Care Plan Study Guide

How to Write Passing Care Plans for the CPNE®

by Sheri Taylor-Jenkins RN, MSN

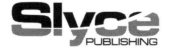
PUBLISHING

Care Plan Study Guide

How to Write Passing Care Plans for the CPNE®

ISBN-13:978-1512246285
ISBN-10:151224628X

Contact Us

4470 Chamblee Dunwoody Rd
STE 450
Atlanta, GA 30338
P- 770.455.8008
F- 770.455.8005
www.atlclinicalworkshop.com

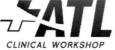

CLINICAL WORKSHOP

Printed in United States of America

Published by

Slyce Publishing

Register Your Care Plan Study Guide

Table of Contents

Foreword

I remember nursing school like it was yesterday and the excitement of going to my clinical and taking care of real patients instead of practicing in the lab. At the same time, I remember the sick feeling in my stomach and the feeling of suffocating because with every patient comes the infamous care plan that was mandatory.

Where was the light bulb that was supposed to be going off in my head? I just didn't get it. I could come up with the diagnostic label and figure out my signs and symptoms but was at a total loss when it came to a rationale or a related to factor. Then just when I thought I was getting close to comprehending this obstacle, out came the red or green marker that my instructor would use to put in her two cents. When trying to challenge what she wrote I knew I was fighting a losing battle because she had co-authored and even written several books and articles of which included care plans.

I kept telling myself to just keep trying and get through school and it would be over. Where was I during the lecture where the instructors told me that I would be care planning for the rest of my nursing career? Even after graduation, the care plans followed me to the NCLEX exam, then to every area of the hospitals I worked in. They were everywhere! That is when I knew I had better face my fears and figure out a way to not only learn them, but to master them. Now, many years later, I want to share my insight with you.

If you ask anyone considering the field of nursing if they know what a care plan is they would probably reply "are you kidding?"

The care plan is one of the most intimidating things for a nursing student to grasp. It does not matter if you are a traditional or non-traditional nursing student, learning to write a solid care plan could be very stressful for you. The goal of this book is to break down the language barrier and explain the care plan process step-by-step in an easy to understand manner.

My goal is to stimulate your brain so you can walk away a little more comfortable with care plans and ready to face that challenge in your nursing career. To lessen your anxiety about writing a care plan I want you to understand that you are constantly care planning even when you are not nursing.

For example, do you write a things to do list? I do, and my list looks something like this:

- ✓ Get up
- ✓ Shower
- ✓ Get ready for work
- ✓ Eat breakfast
- ✓ Check email
- ✓ Straighten house
- ✓ Write checks for bills
- ✓ Mail checks for bills
- ✓ Go to bank and so on…

What are my potential problems? I am needing to complete my ADLs which are required for living but it also cuts down on my stress level knowing they are done. Plus it gives me a sense of accomplishment. Doesn't that sound like a rationale? It is.

What is my goal for that day? To accomplish as many tasks on my list as possible. What are my interventions? Assess my clothes, iron if needed, assess my appearance, brush my hair and teeth, get dressed, assess my bills, write checks for the ones due now, assess my emails and answer the important ones, assess the need to mail the bills before I start my day, drive to the post office to mail the bills, etc… you get my point.

We are constantly doing care plans in our heads we just never looked at it in that way. When I was in traditional nursing school, it was easy for me to understand what I needed to do for the patient and how to set goals for them but for whatever reason, it was also easy for me to have a mental block on care plans. Just the word "care plans" sent me into an anxiety attack it seemed. That was 25 years ago and it has been a mission of mine to find a way to understand care plans then find a way in which to teach them to others so that there is a greater understanding and respect for them by all students.

Not all facilities and programs have the same rules nor teach them the same way but the basic foundations are the same and that is the purpose of this book. It is my goal, as you are reading this book to open your eyes and mind to a better understanding of how to write a care plan based on the rules given to you while preparing for your clinical performance weekend.

What is a Care Plan?

You can find some lively debates on whether or not care plan writing is of any benefit. Some argue that they are a waste of time and not very useful. Others, like myself, argue they are absolutely essential to advance the field of nursing.

Despite your current opinion on the practicality of care plans though, if you're a nursing student you need to know how to write them because you will be given care plan assignments on a regular basis. This is especially true in preparing for your EC clinical weekend.

Care plans are an outline of the nursing care to be provided to a patient. This includes actions the nurse is going to implement to resolve problems identified by an assessment of the patient. This is a guide for ongoing nursing care and assistance in the evaluation of that care. It allows for all nurses taking care of that patient to give continuity of care putting the needs and safety of the patient first. The writing of the care plans is the intermediate stage of the nursing process.

Without a specific document specifying the plan of care, important issues are likely to be neglected. Care planning provides a "road map", to guide all who are involved with a patient care. During your clinical weekend, it is about what you are going to do with your patient. It is your road map to provide the most appropriate treatment that you are assigned in order to ensure the optimal outcome during your time with the patient in the healthcare setting.

Here's a mnemonic to remember what a care plan is.

(Care Plan)
Continuous
Assessment
Review & revise
Everything
Prepare & Plan
Look & listen
Analyze
Never stop

Care Plan Elements

There are 8 essential components of a care plan and every step must be competed before moving onto the next phase of the patient care situation. They are,

1. Finding the appropriate Nanda label

2. Determining the focus for your outcome and only one focus

3. Understanding the physiological ramifications that can occur if you do not fix the problem

4. Knowing what specific assessment you are going to perform to know whether the Nanda problem exists or not

5. Knowing what clinical data from the chart or the nurse report that leads you to the appropriate Nanda label

6. Coming up with two specific interventions that you will perform that will move the patient toward the outcome

7. Understanding the rationale on how the interventions move your patient toward the outcome

8. Knowing who your team members are to request help or advice from

We will go into depth on each section of a care plan but before you can learn to put together a strong care plan you have to be familiar with what phase of the nursing process you are in during your clinical weekend, and I don't mean vaguely familiar. I mean really know and understand the 5 steps of the nursing process because there are certain forms you are required to fill out during the specific areas of the nursing process. The nursing process is the essential core of practice for the registered nurse to deliver holistic, patient-focused care.

Let's take a look at each step of the nursing process.

The Nursing Process

The nursing process is the essential core of practice for the registered nurse to deliver holistic, patient-focused care. The nursing process uses clinical judgment with personal judgment and research evidence to apply critical thinking to take the patient's issues and developing a plan of action. This is an ongoing practice that can end at any stage if the problem is resolved. The nursing process also encompasses the family and community as well as the patient and not only works to fix physiological problems but also on social and emotional needs as well.

Let's take a look at each step of the nursing process.

1. **Assessment.** Collect data from medical record, do a physical assessment of the patient, assess ADLs, look up information about your patient's medical diseases and/or conditions to learn about the signs and symptoms and pathophysiology. For example, a nurse's assessment of a hospitalized patient in pain includes not only the physical causes and manifestations of pain, but the patient's response—an inability to get out of bed, refusal to eat, and withdrawal from family members, anger directed at hospital staff, fear, or request for more pain medication.

2. **Analyze -** Determination of the patient's problem(s)/nursing diagnosis (make a list of the abnormal assessment data, match your abnormal assessment data to likely nursing diagnoses, decide on the nursing diagnoses to use based on your assigned area of care) The nursing diagnosis is the nurse's clinical judgment about the client's response to

actual or potential health conditions or needs. The diagnosis reflects not only that the patient is in pain, but that the pain has caused other problems such as anxiety, poor nutrition, and conflict within the family, or has the potential to cause complications—for example, respiratory infection is a potential hazard to an immobilized patient. The diagnosis is the basis for the nurse's care plan.

3. **Planning.** Write measurable goals/outcomes and nursing interventions. Based on the assessment and diagnosis, the nurse sets measurable and achievable short and long range goals for this patient that might include moving from bed to chair at least three times per day, maintaining adequate nutrition by eating smaller portions, more frequent meals, resolving conflict through counseling or managing pain through adequate medication. Assessment data, diagnosis, and goals are written in the patient's care plan so that nurses as well as other health professionals caring for the patient have access to it. For your clinical weekend, you are going to focus on time spent with your patient only and what your specific assigned areas of care are.

4. **Implementation.** Initiate the care plan. Nursing care is implemented according to the care plan so continuity of care for the patient during hospitalization and in preparation for discharge needs to be assured. Care is documented in the patient's record. Your documentation will be on the Patient Care Situation Response Forms.

5. **Evaluation.** Determine if goals and outcomes have been met. Both the patient's status and the effectiveness of the nursing care must be continuously evaluated and the care plan modified as needed.

The first three steps of the nursing process are tied together during your planning phase on your clinical weekend with each patient you receive. You will observe your assignment written on the kardex, look in the chart and then ask the primary nurse questions to solidify picking priority Nanda labels. You then analyze that data and begin your care planning. In order to do this successfully it is important to understand Nanda labels.

NANDA Labels

Who is NANDA?

NANDA International has approved more than 200 diagnoses for clinical use, testing, and refinement. A nursing diagnosis is "a clinical judgment about individual, family, or community responses to actual or potential health problems/life processes. A nursing diagnosis provides the basis for selection of nursing interventions to achieve outcomes for which the nurse has accountability." (NANDA International, 2009)

Nursing Diagnoses are both actual and potential. For your planning phase, you will be focusing on the actual Nursing Diagnoses. The elements of an actual NANDA-I diagnosis are the label, the definition of the diagnosis, the related factors (causative or associated agents), and the defining characteristics (signs and symptoms.)

Prior to the year 2002, "NANDA" was an acronym for the North American Nursing Diagnosis Association. However, that is no longer the name of the organization. In 2002, they officially became NANDA International and then NANDA International, Inc. in 2011 due to the significant growth of their membership outside of North America. NANDA is still used as part of their name due to the familiarity however it is no longer an acronym for "North American".

There is a Diagnosis Development Committee that formulates and conducts review processes of any proposed diagnoses. The committee has duties such as review of newly proposed labels, proposed revisions, proposed deletions of nursing diagnoses, soliciting and disseminating feedback from experts, implementing processes for review by the membership and voting by the Board of Directors on diagnoses development matters.

Choosing Your NANDA Label

I often get asked the question "How do you know which Nanda to choose?" and that is an open ended question because there are many factors. It is helpful to be familiar with the Nanda labels most commonly used during this specific clinical exam. You can find them in the EC scoring tool. A list of my top 8 are listed in the following section.

You may tab your care plan book as well to the top Nanda labels but you can only write the Nanda name on the tab, nothing else. No hints of any kind can be written on the tab. You may also highlight in your care plan book but no other writing in your book other than your name. Make sure that you have the correct nursing diagnosis book that EC requires.

There are no limitations to using other Nanda labels in your book as long as they are not "risk for", "readiness for", or "health seeking" Nanda labels. The odds of you having to go outside of the top Nanda choices are slim but you do need to be familiar with how to use your book just in case. When you find a Nanda label that you think you might like to use, always read the definition to see if it sounds like your patient. This will save you time and agony trying to make a care plan work and time is not on your side during this exam.

If you understand the nursing process and have a very good care plan book, take a few moments to look at the table of contents page and when you think of a certain Nanda label, read the definition to determine if that sounds like your patient. When I answer care plan questions from students, this sequence is what I keep telling students to follow. Those students who are having problems are not following this sequence of activity. Each care plan begins with a nurse's definition of the diagnosis or main problem. A diagnostic label must be written *word for word*. Any variations or added wording would make this part incorrect, and in turn would make the entire care plan incorrect!

According to NANDA, "nursing diagnosis" is a clinical judgment about individual, family, or community response to an actual or potential health problem(s)/life processes. Nursing interventions are for achieving outcomes for which the nurse is responsible. According to ANA, American Nurses Associate, nursing is the diagnosis and treatment of human responses to actual and potential problems.

Sheri's Top 8 NANDA Choices

Nanda Label	R/T (only pick 1)	Intervention Possibilities
Ineffective airway clearance	Retained secretions	I/S, Cough and deep breathing exercises, position upright
Impaired gas exchange	Ventilation perfusion imbalance/imbalance between oxygen supply and demand	O2 management I/S, cough & deep breathing exercises, position upright
Ineffective breathing pattern	Anxiety/ pain/ musculoskeletal impairment	position upright, administer O2, deep breathe and cough, rest periods
Ineffective peripheral tissue perfusion	Tissue trauma, PVD, CAD, HTN, DM	Musculoskeletal management(AROM, PROM, Movement) PVA, anticoagulants, SCDs, Ted hose
Impaired comfort	Tissue trauma, immobility, disease process, anxiety	Reposition, distraction, guided imagery, massage, face/hand hygiene, straighten linens
Activity intolerance	Bedrest/ generalized weakness/ immobility	Administer O2, assistance with ambulation/reposition AROM/ PROM, rest periods
Impaired physical mobility	Activity intolerance, decreased muscle strength, musculoskeletal impairment	Ambulation/transfer assistance, assistive devices
Dysfunctional gastrointestinal motility	Tissue trauma	Diet, ambulation, reposition, medications that aid in motility

The GRID

What is the GRID?

A GRID is nothing more than a bunch of boxes, twelve to be exact, consisting of four columns and three rows. For this test, a GRID is a plan of action for you! You will have a blank piece of paper somewhere in your packet that you can write this GRID on. Often, students are just putting it on the very back of their packet for the convenience of not flipping through pages.

Each square on the GRID represents how you want to attack this PCS. Give each box a heading then within each square, write out your critical elements, mnemonics, or a things to do list. This will help you keep organized and moving forward without skipping any critical elements.

Writing a GRID

Writing a GRID is simple. Take your blank paper and draw out the 12 boxes in four columns and three rows.

The first five boxes across the top and beginning of second row are the same for all of your patients as well as the last box. You will most likely have to do each of those areas on all assignments so you would only change the specific actions you are told to do and if you are not assigned, then simply put a line through it. For instance one patient you may have to ambulate where another patient you may have to reposition. The headings for the first four boxes are: 1st Thing, 20 Minute

Check, Vital Signs, and Mobility(musculoskeletal management). The last box is always the same which is your Exit box.

The reason we put the first five boxes the same and in that order is because that is the order you should be doing them. At least the first three boxes. After you enter the room then you need to do your 20 minute checks because that is a timed critical element. Then after the 20 minute checks, you want to do the vital signs as quickly as possible. So, in block number three, list *only* the vital signs that you are assigned for your patient. Create a heading for your boxes and within each box is where you will write your mnemonic or your things to do list. Box one is your entry.

Our mnemonic is EWIIG so we would write as follows in box one:

Enter
Wash hands
Introduce self and instructor
ID patient
Grab gloves (is just for convenience because you will need them with your 20 minute check)

Then move onto box 2 and 3. Now box 4 is for mobility/ musculoskeletal management. You don't have to do mobility at this point but it is usually assigned for your pcs so that is why we chose it for the fourth box. In blocks five through ten, you can write the mnemonics for the each of the selected areas of care you are assigned for your specific patient. Personally, medications make sense for the 5th box. If you are not assigned to give medications, you can omit that heading. There is usually a couple of empty blocks on your GRID so use them for any extra notes and don't think you have to fill them all up.

Example: (You may have a different mnemonic .... this is just so you can see what it looks like)

1st Thing	20 Minute Check	Vital Signs	Mobillity
Enter Wash Hands ID patient Introduce self/ instructor Grab pair of gloves	Hydration status IV (rae, amt, type) Palpate site Pump setting Inspect IV tubing Check enteral feeds Oral fluids explain Write down findings Socks on	Temp HR RR BP	Movements Observe alignment Balance/devices Increase support Log response Evaluate
5	6	7	8
9	10	11	**Exit** Side rails up Call light in reach Ask if there is anything else you can do Bed low & locked Say Thank you

We also like to encourage use of colored pens for your GRID. You can write it all in black, but if something has a time limit or is crucial like 0900 meds or fall risk, you may want to write that in red in the appropriate box. Or maybe if you read in the chart that they had shortness of breath with ambulation, you may want to write SOB in green just as a notation that is what you found in the chart. If you do not want to be that obsessive about color coding then you don't have to do that. It is just a suggestion.

I would personally write any assessment findings from the chart or the primary nurse in a different color in the specific box it relates to. It will help you cluster the problems to determine the best Nanda. I would also use a blank box left over to brainstorm possible Nanda labels.

In summary, the GRID is a condensed check off sheet that you create for every patient. It changes with each patient. You also check it and recheck it after every block is completed as a means to check yourself and the work you may have missed. Do not cross into another box without completing everything in the previous box!

Here's a quick recap on using your GRID.

- Do the GRID during the planning phase before turning in your care plan
- As you complete your assignments, check it off on your GRID and make notes of any abnormalities that you need to address in your charting or when giving report to the primary nurse
- Re-check your GRID before you leave the patient's room so you do not miss any critical elements
- Use mnemonics in your GRID to remember your critical elements

Sample Grid

1st Thing in Room	20 Minute Check	Vital Signs	Mobillity
(EWIIG) Enter Wash hands Introduce self ID patient Gloves Safety	(CHIPPICOOOWS) Communicate Hydration status IV (rate, amt, type) Palpate site (gloves) Pump (setting/ drops) Inspect IV tubing Check enteral feeds Oral fluids explain Other drains Oxygen Write down findings Socks on	Temp Pulse Resp BP Weight O2 sat Pain Compare both sets	(RAM SAMS PART) Readiness to learn Assigned areas Morse Fall Scale Strength & support Any Devices & alignment Mobility of joints (appearance/ abnormalities) Symptoms with movement Place Barrier Apply heat/cold Range of motion Traction Evaluate
Meds	**Abdominal Assessment**	**Neuro Assessment**	**Oxygen Management**
(MAR DOSES) MAR check meds Appropriate dose Recheck MAR to ID Do 5 rights Observe allergies Special assessment (BP, pulse) Equipment Sign MAR	(4Ps LLFs RR) Privacy Pee Pain Position Suction Off Look Listen Feel Suction On Reposition Record	(LOGICSS) LOC Observe pupils Grasps (hands) Inspect fontanel Check dorsi flexion Stimuli (noxious) Symmetry of movement (child)	(R SHORT AIRS) Sats Humidity Observe (ears/nares, face, lips, mucous memb., color) Reposition up Tolerance to activity Amount of O2 Ignition sources Reassess and record Sats Post
Possible Nandas	**Other team members**	**Report to Primary**	**Safety/Exit**
M A M M			(SPELLS) Side rails up Phone/call light Everything okay Locked & low bed Lights off/on Say thank you

Mnemonics

What Are Mnemonics?

A mnemonic, from the Greek word *mnemon* meaning mindful (pronounced neh-MAHN-ik) is a memory aid, such as an abbreviation, rhyme or mental image that helps you to remember something. It's a simple shortcut that helps you associate the critical elements for your clinical weekend we want to remember with an image, a sentence, or a word.

Most of the mnemonics that I create are one or two words. With this new edition, they seem to have gotten longer. The fantastic thing about it is that you can get creative with your own mnemonics. The bigger picture here is that you are not struggling to relate to my mnemonics. If they don't work with your memory then please find some that will work for you and your memory style.

A list of all of our mnemonics are in the workshop study guide that you can get in paperback or pdf downloadable version.

Sample Mnemonics

1ST Thing Entering the Room (EWIIGS)

Enter
Wash Hands
Introduce Self
ID patient
Gloves
Safety

20 Minute Check (CHIPPICOOOWS)

Communicate
Hydration status
IV (rate, amount, type)
Palpate site (wear gloves, redness and edema)
Pump (setting/drops)
Inspect tubing (kinks and bubbles)
Check enteral feed
Oral explain
Other drains
Oxygen
Write it down
Socks on

Assessments

Neurological Assessment (LOGICSS)

LOC (person, place, time)
Observe pupils (equal and reactive to light)
Grasp hands (bilaterally)
Inspect fontanel (anterior and upright in 1 year old)
Check dorsi/plantar flexion (bilaterally)
Stimuli (noxious for unconscious pt)
Symmetry of movement (child)

Abdominal Assessment (4Ps LLFs RR)

Privacy
Pee
Pain
Position
Suction off
Look (flat, round, distended,convex, concave AND any drains, incisions, dressings, discoloration)
Listen
Feel (tenderness/pain AND soft/firm/ rigid)
Suction on
Reposition
Record

Managements

Readiness/Patient teaching (with all managements) (LEARN)

Learning readiness
Evaluate knowledge
Act of learning (reading, doing, talking)
Reassess understanding
Need to record

LAIDD (foundation for all patient teachings - alternative to LEARN)

Learn
Assess
Interventions
Determine
Did it work

Comfort Management (AT 2ND CHANCERR)

Assess comfort level using scale (Behaviors, Daisy, Verbal)
Teach
2 Measures
Need to reposition
Distraction
Cold/heat (when assigned)
Hygiene (face/hands or oral/dental)
Arrange linens
Need meds
Comfort rub

Environmental adjustments (lights off/on or temperature)
Relaxation
Re-evaluate and Record

Fluid Management (RAS TRR TRRR)

Readiness
Amount
Site
Type
Rate
Record
Tubing
Residual
Reinstill
Response

IVAD (IVAD TRR)

IV Site & Dressing
Volume
Air/Kinks
Drops/min
Tubing
Rate
Response

D/C an IV (DC CNN)

D/C IV
Dressing applied
Chart CNN
Cannula intact
No active bleeding
No complaints

Enteral Feedings
(FLOW STOMACH R&R)

Feeding type
Low Fowlers
Orient/educate patient
Warmth of solution (room temp)
Select device
Total amount
On time
Monitor feeding during pcs
Assess skin around entry site
Check residual (when assigned)
   (re-instill)
Have baby burp
Reassess/response
Record

HANG NEW SOLUTION
(5 RAS TRTR)

5 Rights
Amount
Site
Type
Rate
Tubing
Record

DRAINAGE/SUCTION
(DRAINAGE MASS ERR)

Drain type/suction type
Response to drain (from pt)
Amount, type, color
Integrity of skin
Need secured (tubing/apparatus)
Assess system (for patency)
Gloves
Empty

Maintain
And
Stabilize or
Secure

Empty - measure
Remove (d/c when assigned)
Record response

Medications
(MAR DOSAGES)

MAR check meds
Appropriate dose
Recheck MAR to ID
Do 5 rights
Observe allergies
Special assessment (BP, pulse, vs, labs)
Ask how patient takes pills
Gather equipment
Evaluate and administer
Sign MAR immediately

Musculoskeletal Management
(RAM SAMS PART)

Readiness to learn
Assigned areas
Morse Fall Scale
Strength and support
Any devices and alignment
Mobility of joints/appearance/ abnormalities
Symptoms with movement (pain, stiffness, etc.)
Place Barrier
Apply heat/cold (when assigned)
Range of motion (when assigned)
Traction

Mobility
(MOBILE)

Movements
Observe alignment
Balance/devices
Increase support
Log response
Evaluate

Oxygen Management
(R PASS CC SAFERS)

Readiness to learn
Position upright
Amount of O2 verify (during 20 min check)
Sats
Safety/ignition/tubing
Color
Clubbing
Skin Integrity of ears/nares/face (lips, mucous membranes, skin)
Activity intolerance
Flow of humidity
Effort of breathing
Reassess and record
Sats

"OR"

(R SHORT AIRS)

Readiness
Sats
Humidity
Observe skin (color, nares, ears, face, lips, mucus membranes)
Reposition up
Tolerance to activity (shortness of breath)

Amount of O2
Ignition sources/ safety
Report color/clubbing
Sats post

Peripheral Neurovascular Management
(R PERIPH ME HOT MESSED)

Readiness
Pulses
Extremity
Refill
Is sensation
Pale/pink
Hot/cold
Motor function
Edema
Help
Offer blanket
Two
Movement/reposition
Exercise
SCDs
Stockings
Evaluate
Document

Respiratory Management
(RUBBERSS ROAR)

Readiness
Upright
Bare skin
Breathe
Effort (rate, rhythm, depth)
Receptacle
Sats
Secretions

I/S
DB&C
Reassess what learned
Oral care
Assess sats again
Record

SUCTION
Trach (ESS SOBS 15)

Explain
Sats
Suction
Breathe
15 sec
Sats

Oral (ESS B 15)

Explain
Sats
Suction
Breathe
15 sec

Bulb (DIA)

Deflate
Insert
Aspirate

Skin Management
(Braden R SKINNED OPARKA)

Braden scale
Readiness to learn
Skin color
Keep warm/dry (check temp)
Integrity intact
Note edema
Need repositioned
Evaluate pain
Do 1 area (2 interventions)
Observe turgor
Provide incontinent care
Apply/maintain devices
Reposition
Keep skin clean
Apply protective products (barrier)

Wound Management
(OUCH WOUNDED SKIN)

Observe behavior
U ready
Check pain
Have nurse medicate
Wound location
Observe drainage/type/appearance
Unique irrigation and supplies
Need clean or sterile?
Dressing change
Evaluate pain and tolerance
Dispose in appropriate receptacle
Secure dressing
Keep skin, clothes, linens dry
Initial date and time
Note

IRRIGATION
(STOP FLOW)

Solution
Temperature of solution
Other equipment
Position
Flow rate
Linens dry
Observe tolerance
Write down

Exit
(SPELLS)

Side rails up
Phone/call light in reach
Everything ok
Locked and low bed
Lights off/on
Say thank you

Exit/Safety Pedi Patient
(CRYS)

Crib rails up
Reach (infant/child should be in
  reach when side rails down)
You see (infant/child should be in
  sight during care)
Secure the infant/child when out of
  bed in seat/chair

Other options for Exit mnemonics
(CALL DONE)

Call light
Anything else
Locked
Lights
Do side rails
Other items in reach
Non skid socks
Everything okay

(BECAUSE)

Bed low and locked
Educate on:
Call light
All personal items in reach
Up on rails
Socks on
Everything okay

(BURPS)

Bed low and locked
Use call light
Rails up
Personal items in reach
Say thank you

(BRACESS)

Bed low and locked
Rails up
All items in reach
Call light
Everything okay
Socks
Say thank you

Writing a Care Plan

Structuring Your Care Plan

There are a couple of components to the structure of the care plan. First, you have the Nanda label and secondly, you have the Nanda diagnostic statement. The diagnostic statement consists of telling the story of what the problem is, what caused that problem, and how you know the problem exists. When you begin to write your care plans during your planning phase, the Nanda label is what you are concerned with and what caused the problem not the entire statement. We will get into the entire statement later.

The Nanda label is the problem that exists. The labels in your care plan books are the actual problems unless the words "risk for" are in front of the label. If the words "risk for" are in front of the Nanda label, those are not permissible to use during the planning phase. The Nanda labels you want to choose are ones that are actual problems that are currently occurring with your patient based on what you are assigned to do. If you *think* a problem *might* exist but you are not sure then it is a "risk for" care plan or a "potential problem" and you will not get your foot in the door during your clinical. You are no longer allowed to use acute pain, chronic pain and definitely no "readiness' or "health seeking" Nanda labels.

If the Nanda label is the problem that exists, how do you know it exists if you are writing the care plan before you get into the room and see your patient? You are getting information from the chart over the last 24 hours and asking questions to the primary nurse or examiner. This gives you just enough leeway to formulate a care plan or a plan of action until you get into the room and observe those signs and symptoms yourself.

A nursing diagnostic statement consists of writing the Nanda label, the related to (which is the etiology or the cause of the problem) and the aeb (as evidenced by or signs and symptoms.) During your planning phase, it does not ask for the aeb. This comes at the end of your patient care situation during the evaluation phase and is written on the evaluation form.

The Nanda label is the only thing that must be written word for word. There should be no misspellings or rewording. There is no need for that because all you are doing is simply copying it right out of your care plan book. Probably the most common mistake I have seen in my 12 years of teaching people how to pass their clinical weekend is Ineffective Peripheral tissue perfusion. Many students leave off the word "peripheral" and that would constitute a fail. Another mistake is Dysfunctional gastrointestinal motility. I have often seen students write "mobility" instead of motility. Whether it is nerves or moving too fast through the test, it is a careless mistake that could cost you your nursing license in the real world so please be conscientious to what you are doing.

Flow of the Planning Phase

When you receive your assignment, the pcs assignment sheet will be filled out and all other forms will be blank unless you are giving meds, then the MAR will be filled out as well. You are only to write on the plan of care form and you can put your GRID on any blank page that you have available. We encourage that you immediately highlight your assignments. Then look in the chart for pertinent information, like the most recent nurses notes, to see what problems occurred the previous shift. Look at baseline vitals or even the progress notes from the doctor because that can let you know what the plans are for that patient. Also look at the orders to see if anything new has been written. Take notes. You can make notes on your pcs assignment sheet, on a blank piece of paper, or on your GRID. Write your GRID in pen (even use colors) and care plans in black pen.

Your next step is to create you GRID. Color code the GRID if you would like. Look for any unanswered areas that you can ask questions to your primary nurse if need be. For this exam, your examiner will probably step in as the primary nurse in the beginning to answer any questions. Remember that you cannot ask the primary nurse/examiner any how-to questions.

Here is where you follow the acronym MAMM! This is simply the order of looking at your assignments and brainstorming all possible Nanda labels based on your assignment. We have also made box 9 on your GRID to write your MAMM and your Nanda labels.

Immediately go to the managements first because that is where you have more interventions to do for your patient. Ask yourself, "Does the patient have an actual problem with this management that I am assigned?" If not, move on to your next management that you are assigned or if no other managements are assigned, move to your assessment assigned and ask the same question. If the answer is yes, keep moving onto the next step. What Nanda labels might go with this problem? Start thinking about the most commonly used Nanda labels and write them in box 9 of your GRID. If you have your nursing diagnosis book tabbed with the Nanda labels, you can simply start looking at your tabs to see if one triggers your memory.

Once you go through all of your managements, and ask yourself if they actually have a problem then make a list of all possible Nanda labels and put in box 9 on your GRID. Now, according to Maslows, which Nanda label in that list should be your priority to focus on? Once you figure that out, go to your plan of care form and write your Nanda down.

Look up the Nanda in your care plan book and read the definition of that Nanda. If this sounds like your patient, keep going and write down the Nanda in the Nanda box (3rd box) on your plan of care form. I recommend that you put the page number in the margin on the left of the plan of care form in case you need to look it up later on in your diagnosis book and are rushing or nervous. If you are having trouble coming up with a Nanda label, you can look up the medical diagnosis in section I of the Mosby's diagnosis handbook and see what it suggests, but always refer to section II of Mosby's to write your care plan. Other diagnosis books may have this option as well. If you are following my top 8, you should know them by heart by the time you go test.

The next step is to look at what assessment findings from the chart or the primary nurse/examiner that led you to assume that this is a true problem. This is where writing those findings in green on my GRID where it fits helps. That is the first two boxes on the plan of care form. The heading says assessment but it does not mean that is the assessment you are going to do but rather the assessment finding that leads you to believe this Nanda is a problem. If you think about it, the chart and the primary nurse are your eyes and ears in the planning phase until you can go into the room yourself and see what is really going on for you.

I like to tell students to write the Nanda label first on the plan of care form. Everything should focus around that Nanda so it keeps the perspective going. So write your Nanda in the 3rd box, then go to box 1 and 2 and list your assessment findings from the chart or the primary nurse that lead you to that Nanda.

The 4th box on the plan of care form is the rationale for why you picked the nursing diagnosis. This should be focused on

Maslow's Hierarchy of Needs and specific to your patient. It should also have a couple of complications that can occur if you don't fix the problem.

Some ideas for physiological complications that can occur:

- Pneumonia, atelectasis
- Hypoxia, confusion, or altered mental status
- Decreased GI motility, constipation, bowel obstruction, peritonitis, ileus
- DVTs, pulmonary embolisms

The 5th box is the related factor. In your Mosby's book, there is a heading under each specific label that says related factors. It is simply what cause the problem. You can read the options your book gives you and pick the one that fits what is going on with your patient. You can also use a medical diagnosis that the patient has.

For example, if you choose Ineffective airway clearance, the related factor could be retained secretions (which is a suggestion in your Mosby's book) or it could be Pneumonia or Bronchitis if that is your patient's medical diagnosis.

The 6th box is the expected patient outcome.

The Outcome

The outcome needs to be written in a manner that answers three questions: who is doing it, what specifically they are doing and during what time frame. It must be very precise, clear, and measurable. The interventions that you're choosing to do for the care plan must also move the patient toward the outcome chosen. Ideas for outcomes are in your care plan books but they are vague so you have to make them specific to your patient.

It is important to remember that the outcome is the goal you have in mind for the patient to achieve while you are with them. It also leads you to the evaluation of whether the patient achieved it or not. The outcome needs to also match your chosen diagnosis and that is where it helps to look for options in your care plan book. Avoid vague words for your outcome like "adequate", "normal", "increased", "decreased", "less", or "adequate". For outcome, it has to be the maximum best outcome for the patient so you wouldn't say "less red" instead you should say there would be "no redness." Besides, "less" is subjective.

An outcome cannot sound like an intervention. If you chose Impaired physical mobility for your Nanda and your outcome said patient will ambulate in room x 1 with a steady gait during pcs, your intervention could not say ambulate patient in room. They are too much alike. You could say assist with ambulation if you were told to do so or encourage patient to ambulate if that is what you are told but make sure the wording is not identical. The interventions are what you are going to do to move the patient toward the outcome.

If lung sounds are in the assessment, then lung sounds has to be in the outcome and the evaluation for the as evidenced by or the signs and symptoms. Use "same terms" throughout the nursing care plan.

For example, if you want to focus on Ineffective airway clearance and the assessment is auscultate the lung sounds then your outcome should look like this: The patient/client will have clear lung sounds in upper and lower lobes bilaterally after interventions or during the pcs.

The first care plans you do take the longest. This is a new skill you are learning and it is a bit complex only because you have to keep so many things in your mind. Commit to them on paper to help you out so you don't lose track of what is going on.

Tips for Your Outcome

- It is usually opposite of your Nanda label or the signs and symptoms (AEB)
- Time frame needs to focus on your time during the pcs. It could be by discharge but is really great if you can focus on short term goals that you are able to re-evaluate during your time with your patient.
- Do not use the direct outcome from your diagnosis book. You may use it as a guide for the idea but must be specific to your patient and measurable.
- Statement needs to be very specific…must see it (observe; patient will do), hear it (patient will verbalize), feel it (eg… temperature)
- It is only *one* thing; one focus….using the word "and" in an outcome statement makes it more than one outcome/focus so figure out which one you want to use.
- This is what you expect the patient to achieve "after" you perform your interventions
- It is okay if your outcome is not met during your time with the patient but it needs to be something that could possibly be achieved during that time
- Don't use vague words like: appropriate, adequate, normal, etc… be specific
- Don't use the statement patient will have "less"……. How do you measure "less"? Again, specific…no edema, no redness, not less. The only time you can use "less" is if they verbalize it.
- Outcomes need a time frame like during pcs or after interventions
- Do not abbreviate unless it is an approved abbreviation and that is just too much added info to put into your already overwhelmed brain.
- Cannot sound like an intervention

- Look at each problem and ask the question, "Will this problem get better?" (Or, "Can we make this problem better?") If the answer is yes, then your goal will be for the problem to resolve or show signs of improvement within the review period.
- If the problem is not likely to improve, then another question you want to ask yourself is "what can I do to maintain or provide optimal quality of life, comfort, and dignity for this person."
- In summary, the outcome must be specific and tell who is going to achieve it, what are they going to achieve and during what time frame.

Your nursing diagnosis book has some ideas but remember that the book is very vague and is designed to be a guideline. The nursing diagnosis book was not written specifically for your school or organization so you have a little bit of work to do and must follow the rules for your school requirements.

The 7th box has a #1 and is for your first intervention.

The 8th box is the rationale for why you picked the first intervention and how it moves the patient toward the outcome you have chosen.

The 9th box has a #2 and is for your second intervention.

The 10th box is the rationale for why you picked the second intervention and how it moves the patient toward the outcome you have chosen.

The Interventions

Interventions are actions that you are *already assigned* to do that will move the patient toward the outcome. This is really one of the hardest things that I find for students to grasp which is why I encourage writing a GRID first. The GRID helps because it is listing your assignments (interventions) in each box so you can refer quickly to the boxes and find actions you can do.

Often, you will hear me refer to "Simon Says" and only do what Simon Says. The interventions *are* your critical elements. Don't think outside of the box or over think the situation. It is not about what interventions you would do for a specific diagnosis or what you normally do at work. Instead it is being able to do what you are assigned *only*. What are you going to do and, if you do this, will it help to move the patient toward the outcome?

Now does this mean that you cannot come up with other interventions to do that you were not assigned? No, it doesn't. However, if you rely on your GRID or your plan of care form, those interventions that you were not assigned to do are not going to be there and you just might forget to chart it in your narrative notes. So if you chose to do this, please don't forget to write those extra interventions down on your GRID to keep you from omitting anything.

Interventions cannot be assessments. Some students try to manipulate their wording like saying palpate the abdomen or auscultate bowel sounds, etc… which sounds like you are really doing something for the patient but it is only giving you data. Assessments do nothing for the patient. So no using words like assess, observe, inspect, etc. You will see in your Mosby's book that there are many assessment options for interventions in there but keep in mind that the Mosby's book or any other Nanda book was not written specifically for you and your school's requirements and you have to follow the rules for your school. It is just a guideline for you.

Tips for Interventions

- Must be actions therefore contain action words
- Must be effective in moving the patient toward the outcome
- Some action words: instruct, encourage, administer, provide, offer, continue to administer
- Must be done during the time with your patient
- Both interventions cannot be administration of medication so if you have two medications that you are assigned to give, pick the one that will work during your pcs
- There are interventions listed in your diagnosis book as well but when you find an intervention that you think you might like to use then look at your GRID and see if you are assigned or going to be doing during your pcs
- Remember: Ice or Heat must be assigned and stays on for 15 minutes with a barrier in place
- Repositioning is an overlapping intervention. If you are not assigned, but it needs to be done, you can use it
- When you are struggling to find interventions, it might be a sign to find another Nanda label
- Don't abbreviate
- Highlighting interventions in your NANDA book helps so you don't get hung up or mixed up searching around when you are trying to write your care plan in a hurry.
- Use words like encourage or assist, you can also use "teaching" type words.
- Physically doing something= perform or administer

Intervention Problems

- Administer medications as ordered (how are they ordered? Be specific and only pick one med.
- Administer IV fluids as ordered (how are they ordered? Be specific)

- Maintain bed rest is not so much of an action. Would be better to "encourage" bed rest but even better would be to assist with reposition.
- Maintain hip in proper alignment, using a triangular abduction pillow (you could not use the abduction pillow unless told to on your pcs assignment form)
- Reposition the patient frequently (what is frequently? How often were you told to reposition? Remember you are only with the patient for a short while and interventions should be what you are assigned to do)
- Encourage frequent coughing and deep-breathing exercises (what is frequent? Avoid vague words and do what were you assigned to do?)
- Assess for complications, such as infection and abnormal bleeding (no assessments for interventions)
- Consult with physical therapy (no consulting. Remember you are only the student in an unfamiliar facility). There is a spot for promotion of teamwork.
- Arrange for rehabilitation as appropriate (no consulting of outside resources) as an intervention.
- Give anticoagulation therapy as ordered (how is it ordered? Be specific)

Promotion of Teamwork

The next page of your plan of care form asks you to specify task/care to be performed and to identify the team member to perform the task/care. This is puzzling to students but is really simple. Let's say that you are not assigned to ambulate the patent but that you know they are allowed to ambulate. Who would you get to ambulate the patient? Would it be physical therapy? The UAP or tech? So the task would be ambulate and the team member would be whomever is assigned to do it.

Another example would be output. If you were not assigned output but the patient needs to go to the restroom, if you are allowed to ambulate them to the bathroom but not assigned to manage the output, who is? The UAP? So the task would be measure/record the output and the person would be the UAP.

Once you are finished with the Initial POC (Plan of Care) and have filled out all 10 boxes and the promotion of teamwork section, you then hand in your paperwork to be graded. Make sure that first column is completely filled out with no blanks.

After it is graded, they will not say "good job." They will simply say "you are now ready to enter the implementation phase." Remember the nursing process? AAPIE or ADPIE? They are following the nursing process. This means you are going into the room and going to start working from your GRID and get your assignments done.

Revisions

Sometimes you will have to revise your care plan. Revisions of a care plan should not intimidate you. It is simply correcting particular aspects of your previously written care plan or, in some cases, writing another care plan. Keep in mind that revising a care plan, or having to rewrite one, doesn't mean that you have done something irreversibly wrong. It's just an opportunity to correct a weak care plan that could have cost you in the long run.

Some reasons to revise your care plan are,

- When your Nanda label is no longer an actual problem
- If your interventions are not carried out (for whatever reason)
- If the intervention does not move the patient toward the outcome

- If the problem or outcome has already been resolved before you implement anything

When you are in the room taking care of your patient and you discover for whatever reason that the care plan needs adjusting:

- Figure out what you need to change
- Make corrections with the patient (example, if the patient refuses an intervention, try to find another intervention to take its place and implement it before revising to make sure they will do it)
- Simply tell the examiner that you want to make a clinical decision to revise your care plan and explain why. Step out and complete the Revised Plan of Care section on your Plan of Care form
- You only revise once

In the planning phase, you cannot have a risk for care plan. During the revision phase, you should still have an actual problem not a risk for. A risk for care plan does not have an aeb or signs and symptoms because it is only a potential problem that could occur. It is not recommended that the risk for care plan be taken into the evaluation phase.

Revised POC

- Boxes 1 and 2 are for new assessment findings if they were not the same as what you read in the chart or information received from the primary nurse/examiner. If they are the same, leave those blank.
- Nanda box is only filled out if you changed your Nanda label.
- Rationale for the selected nursing diagnosis is only filled out in this section if you changed your Nanda label.
- Expected outcome box is filled out if that is the part of the revision you are changing. If you did not change your outcome, leave it blank.

- Nursing Intervention 1 box is to be filled out only if that is the intervention you are changing.
- Rationale for intervention 1 is filled out when you revise the intervention and is the same as in the planning phase, you are prioritizing according to Maslow and explaining why it is important, how it relates to your patient, and what complications can occur if you do not fix the problem.
- Nursing Intervention box 2 is filled out only if that is the intervention you are changing
- Rationale for intervention 2 is filled out when you revise the intervention and is the same as in the planning phase, you are prioritizing according to Maslow and explaining why it is important, how it relates to your patient, and what complications can occur if you do not fix the problem.
- The final thing to fill out during a revision is on the next page, below the promotion of teamwork it says "reason for revision." The reason you gave the examiner in the room is the very thing you write in this section

Are you lost yet? If you are not familiar with the forms in your appendix A of your EC study guide, you need to get familiar with them. I would suggest that if you have not done so, print out appendix A and have it beside you while reading this book and make notes and find the form or heading that I am talking about when you are reading this. Also, with the online workshop, in the care plan videos, I go through writing the grid, the steps through the plan of care process, revision process, and evaluation process so if you need additional support be sure to check that out. Visit our website www.atlclinicalworkshop.com.

The Evaluation Phase

The evaluation phase is the last part of the nursing process and at the end of your care plan. You use your revised care plan at this point if you did a revision.

You know how in the planning phase, you were thinking "how do I know what problem the patient has if I have not had the opportunity to see them yet?" Now, you have had the opportunity to get into the room and work with your patient, assessing what is going on and fixing problems. The first two boxes are what assessment findings you actually found that go with your Nanda. Huh? You say. Let's say that you read in the chart your patient was not taking deep breaths and they have rhonchi in their bases so that is your assessment findings in the planning phase. Once you got into the room and you assessed your patient, is that the same thing you found? If it is you put the findings in box 1 and box 2 of the evaluation phase. If you found something different then you would put what you found.

The next box, are boxes that ask if your outcome was met, partially met, or not met. Remember that I said earlier it is okay not to meet your outcome. Simply check the box that applies.

Final box is an evaluation of how those interventions you did worked to move the patient toward the outcome. If you said the patient will have clear lung sounds in upper and lower lobes bilaterally after interventions, did they? If they did you would say "after interventions, lung sounds were found to be clear in upper and lower lobes bilaterally."

If it is partially met or not met, will continuing those interventions eventually help the patient or should you have revised to some other intervention? If they will help then after you check the box partially met or not met, write that statement "after interventions, the patient's lung sounds remain with rhonchi in the lower bases" however "continuation of these interventions will eventually move the patient to the outcome chosen.

Always specify that the interventions need to continue if you partially met or did not meet the outcome. What you are saying is hey, we can't discontinue the treatment because we are not at goal yet.

The evaluation phase is where your documentation is to be thorough enough to show your effectiveness of all of the interventions you have done. You will need to determine if you did what you said you were going to do and if you did not, then why and were you able to meet the expectations of your goals.

16 Step Care Plan Checklist

1. Read the patient information.
2. Write down what categories you are in charge of on your GRID.
3. Look at your managements on your GRID. Do they tie into the patient's problems?
4. Use the mnemonics for the categories you are in charge of to know what actions you need to take with the patient. (Those actions ARE your INTERVENTIONS.)
5. Turn to that diagnostic label you have chosen.
6. Read the definition of the Nanda. Does your patient have this problem?
7. Read the signs and symptoms in your book, which are listed as defining characteristics.
8. Ask yourself "Do any of these match my patient's signs and symptoms?" based on the chart findings or info from the primary nurse or examiner
9. If yes, read the interventions.
10. Ask yourself, "Do any of these interventions match what I'm assigned to do on my PCS assignment?"
11. Write the diagnostic label down.
12. Write down the two assessment findings that lead you to this Nanda label (this is in your Mosby's book under defining characteristics if you need help but should come from the chart or the primary nurse).
13. Write down your reason for picking the Nanda

14. The next part of your statement is the related to. Ask yourself "what is making me think this patient has this problem?" That is your related to. You can use a medical diagnosis!

15. Write the outcome statement or goal for your patient. (It should be opposite of your problem and it should be something you can measure during your PCS.)

16. Now write down your two interventions you will use that will move the patient toward the outcome and that you are assigned to already do.

Rules to Care Planning

Assessments
- Not what assessments you are going to do
- Findings from the chart or primary nurse/examiner that *lead* you to the Nanda

Nanda Label
- Must be written word for word (no misspells or alteration in any way)
- No risk for
- No acute or chronic pain
- No readiness for or health seeking

Related Factor
- R/T cannot be surgery, surgical procedure or a person
- It is what is causing the problem
- Can be a medical diagnosis

Outcome
- Outcomes are vague in Mosby's so make them measurable
- Interventions and outcomes cannot have the same wording

Interventions
- One single, specific intervention that MOVES the patient toward the outcome
- No Assessments for interventions
- No referrals to other resources
- Interventions are about what you are going to do

Common Care Plan Questions

There are many common questions I'm asked about writing a care plan. Here are some great questions full of important nuggets of information that will help you write a stronger care plan every time. These are in no particular order and are all equally as valuable to your care planning skills for your clinical weekend.

What part of the diagnostic statement has to be written word for word?

The Nanda label is the only thing in your Mosby's book that must be written word for word because the label was created by NANDA-I, voted in by a panel and not allowed to be altered in any way.

Where do you find the r/t in your Mosby's book?

The related to is in the Mosby's book under the specific Nanda label and the related factors heading. This is what is causing the problem or also called the etiology and this can be altered to be specific to your patient.

Where do you find the aeb (as evidenced by) in your Mosby's book?

The as evidenced by, or AEB, is found in the Mosby's book under the specific Nanda label and defining characteristics heading. The aeb is a sign and symptom of the Nanda and you will not know it until you get into the room and actually see the patient. However, the as evidenced by IS the two assessment findings you got from the chart or primary nurse in the planning phase! Your AEB is not required on your planning phase form but rather on your evaluation form under the #1 and #2 assessments on the evaluation part on the Plan of Care form.

Where do you find the interventions in your Mosby's book?

The interventions are found in the shaded boxes in the Mosby's book under each Nanda label. Remember that even though an intervention is in the Mosby's book, it does not make it okay to use it. (This is crucial to grasp.) You cannot use an assessment for an intervention on your care plan.

What are reasons to revise your care plans?

When you realize the problem no longer exists, you would need to revise it. All interventions must be carried out with your patient. If an intervention has been refused or the order has changed and that intervention is no longer needed then you would also have to revise. It is okay for the outcome not to be met so that does not need a revision. The only time the outcome is considered for revision is if you want to change the focus. For example, if you used "patient will have palpable, strong, and equal pedal pulses bilaterally" and they already do but they have cold feet, then you would revise your outcome to the patient will have warm feet bilaterally.

How do you prioritize for your care plans?

Tricky question. You are first basing your Nanda labels on what you are assigned and how that assignment ties into the patient's problems based on your findings in the chart or from the primary nurse. Once you have several Nanda labels picked out, you prioritize according to Maslow's to come up with your top two Nanda labels.

Do you have to use a GRID?

A GRID is not necessary according to EC. However, we encourage it and have seen it be the golden nugget to keep you focused during your test so you have all of your critical elements together in one spot. It is usually placed on a blank form in your pcs packet or some will put it on the very back of the packet.

What is the main reason for the GRID?

The purpose of a GRID is organization and to keep you on track during your pcs. Even though your pcs assignment is filled out with your assignments, your critical elements are not listed so how are you going to remember your critical elements when you are in the room and nervous? Mnemonics are very helpful but where are you going to write them? That is where a GRID comes into play. Keeping you organized and focused cuts down on fails.

Can you highlight in your Mosby's book?

Highlighting is acceptable in your Mosby's book. It is clearly expressed in your EC study guide that you are allowed to highlight. It is not cheating when you are highlighting something that is already in print. It is considered a visual jogger.

Can you write in your Mosby's book?

The only thing that can be written in your Mosby's book is your name. No notes can be written in your book. It would be considered academic dishonesty if you do and they will pick up your book and thumb through it looking for writing.

Can you tab your Mosby's book?

Tabbing of your Mosby's book is allowed. The only thing you can write on your tabs is the Nanda label. No medical diagnoses on the tabs. I like to color code my tabs so any respiratory Nanda labels are blue, Circulation or Mobility and Pain labels are red, and GI, urinary, Deficient fluid volume etc. with green labels. Just an idea.

What are good examples of assessment on the initial plan of care? Trick question? It depends on your Nanda that you chose. Example, for Ineffective Airway Clearance:

Rhonchi, wheezes, rales

Weak cough

Short of breath

You are assigned vital signs with 0-10 pain scale and comfort management for a patient with sickle cell who is rating pain a 6 in their legs. Which Nanda labels would you pick?

Acute pain nor chronic pain cannot be used anymore as a Nanda choice. You were assigned comfort management therefore Impaired comfort should be your focus on the planning phase form as long as you have assessment findings that prove the patient is uncomfortable. A rule of thumb, if assigned comfort management you go with Impaired comfort. When pain assessment is with vital signs, they have not assigned you to manage pain.

Can you use teaching as an intervention?

Teaching is a wonderful thing and now you are required to teach with all of your managements so on your pcs assignment you may not see it worded to specifically teach but you have to know it is a critical element. To answer this question, absolutely! Words to describe could be teach, instruct, encourage, or educate.

Do Interventions have to be in Mosby's book?

It is safer if you match up your assignments/interventions on your pcs assignment or in your critical elements with those listed in the shaded boxes in your care plan book. What if the examiner asks you to show them where you got that intervention? Will you have something to show them if you did not find it in the book? No. So at that point, you are going to have to explain your way out of that. It can be done but they do not have to accept the intervention you chose if they don't feel like the intervention moves the patient toward the outcome.

Where will items like splints, trochanter rolls, traction, side rails be found on the pcs assignment?

Those will be specific under musculoskeletal management and the side rails would be listed under safety. When you have some extra time, pick apart your pcs assignment and look at the areas that have lines beside the caption for something to be written on them and review that section of your study guide to see what types of things the examiners can write there.

Why is it that we cannot use assessments for interventions?

Interventions are actions that you are going to perform that will move the patient toward the outcome. If you ask yourself "if I do this then will it move the patient toward the outcome," your answer will always be *no* for an assessment therefore it cannot be used.

Why is it that you cannot use a "risk for" care plan in the planning phase?

During the planning phase, you need to find actual problems that are occurring with this patient. Even though you have not seen the patient yet, looking in the chart and asking the primary nurse questions will lead you to knowing what problems are currently existing. You are only required to come up with one care plan and it should be actual.

What is not allowed to be used for a r/t?

The related to is what is causing a problem. It can be a medical diagnosis. It is best to be a nursing problem instead of a medical diagnosis but a medical diagnosis is okay. What is not okay is when you relate the problem to a surgery or surgical procedure or a person because then it sounds like you are blaming the person or the procedure and having a procedure is a good thing and a person helping you is a good thing. The r/t is the cause. So don't blame a person or a procedure.

What if the CE assigns respiratory management with deep breathing and coughing and I/S x 5 but CE tells you that the patient's lung sounds are clear?

If you observe in the chart or receive report that breath sounds are clear, it does not matter if you are assigned respiratory management or not, they don't have a problem. If they don't have a problem, you don't address it in the planning phase. But you DO still have to perform the management. Now, once you get into the room, if you feel like airway clearance is still an important focus even though there are no current problems, you can revise to a risk for care plan but you would be changing your entire care plan because you would not have entered the room with Ineffective airway clearance as your Nanda.

If the order says for patient to perform I/S x5 and I put that on my care plan, but when I get into the room the patient can only do 2, do I have to revise my care plan?

The interventions are to be carried out in the room. If you attempted to carry out the intervention and the patient partially did them, did it move the patient toward the outcome? If the answer is *yes* even though they only did two, then you would not have to revise your care plan.

How do I write an outcome for Impaired skin integrity?

When you choose the Nanda Impaired skin integrity, you should be focusing on an area that is red, blanched, or more superficial and the outcome would be best if focused on the redness. An example for this would be "the patient will have no redness to the gluteal area during the pcs."

Common Care Plan Mistakes

"Learn all you can from the mistakes of others. You won't have time to make them all yourself." -Alfred Sheinwold

Through grading hundreds of care plans every week for EC students I've noticed many reoccurring mistakes students make time and time again. Making mistakes is inevitable when you're learning to write care plans for your clinical weekend. What's important is that you learn from them. Even better though, is not making them at all because you've learned from the mistakes of others. Pay close attention because any one of these tips could save you from turning in a failing care plan.

Here's what not to do...

X **sing a surgery or surgical procedure like hysterectomy for a r/t or related factor.** The r/t or related factor is what is causing the problem. It cannot be a surgery, surgical procedure, or a person. Just because you don't put the word "surgery" in the statement, does not give you the okay to use the medical terminology word for the surgery.

X **Describing lung sounds as "regular" or "normal" for an outcome.** Breath sounds are either clear, rhonchi, wheezes, or rales. They are not just abnormal for this test. When writing an outcome, it has to be very specific, clear and concise, as well as measurable. The best way to write an outcome for lung sounds is to say "the patient will have clear lung sounds in upper and lower lobes bilaterally after interventions during the pcs."

✗ **Using the word "maintain" in the outcome.** Whenever we use the word "maintain" in a statement that means they are already doing it. So if you write "maintain clear lung sounds," that means the patient already has clear lung sounds which changes the meaning of your care plan to a risk for and not an actual problem. You are not allowed to write risk for care plans during the planning phase.

✗ **Using "range of motion" in an intervention when not assigned.** When we write range of motion as an intervention, we have to say whether it is upper or lower and whether it is passive or active range of motion. It also must be assigned and you would see it marked on your pcs assignment under musculoskeletal management.

✗ **Saying "perform range of motion to prevent contractures" for an intervention.** Range of motion must be assigned but when it is assigned you have to say active or passive, to upper or lower and interventions should not explain why you are doing it. They are only looking for the action not the explanation. Now the box just below the intervention is where you put why it will help.

✗ **Saying "maintain IV fluids" for an intervention.** If you are in charge of IV fluids that is fine but when writing the intervention you need to state the name of the fluid and what rate it is running at. Remember that you have to be very specific in the statement of what you are doing for your intervention.

✗ **Using "deep breathing" as one intervention and "have patient cough" as a second intervention.** Deep breathing and coughing is one intervention and is not to be split up. You will need an additional intervention that will also move the patient toward the outcome you have chosen. Often positioning upright or incentive spirometry are good choices.

✗ **Saying "provide rest periods before ambulation" for activity intolerance.** Providing rest periods is a good intervention but if they have already been in bed prior to ambulation haven't they already been resting? Maybe provide rest periods during ambulation.

✗ **Writing an outcome for Impaired tissue integrity saying "the patient will have no breakdown during pcs."** With Impaired tissue integrity, the outcome usually focuses on drainage so you would say "the patient will have no drainage to the _____(region) during the pcs."

✗ **Administering two medications for interventions.** Administration of a medication is one intervention so you pick the medication that will have the biggest impact during your pcs.

✗ **Not putting "during pcs" on the outcome.** The outcome must tell who is going to do it, what they are going to do, and over what time frame. The time frame should be during the pcs or after interventions.

✗ **Not writing the Nanda label word for word.** This is the easiest thing to do yet one of the most common reasons for failing and not even get into the room. All you do is find the Nanda you wish to use and simply copy it from your Mosby's book.

✗ **Not writing a specific assessment.** The two assessments are specific assessment findings that you found in the chart or from the primary nurse that you are going to proves whether the Nanda problem exists or not.

✗ **Using nonskid socks for a mobility intervention.** Nonskid socks are a necessity and a safety measure but according to EC, they do not make the patient actually walk therefore you cannot use nonskid socks as an intervention for any of the mobility Nanda labels.

✗ **Saying "position upright at 30 or 45 degrees" for an intervention.** The actual degrees for positioning a patient upright are 90 degrees so saying 30 or 45 degrees and upright in the same sentence does not even make sense and is incorrect. Either specify a degree or say position upright but not both in the same sentence. And for auscultating breath sounds they need to be at a 90 degree angle in order to be able to get to the proper landmarks so 30 or 45 degrees would still be incorrect if you choose an outcome about breath sounds.

✗ **Requesting the primary nurse to medicate.** Requesting they medicate with what? You need to be specific on the medication and you need to make sure that they do in fact get medicated during your time with the patient. The problem is that when you are assigned pain management, the examiners are expecting you to personally do something to help the patient's pain improve. Notifying the primary nurse to medicate is not you doing anything so to me that should be a last resort.

✗ **Saying "patient will have normal bowel sounds" for an outcome.** Bowel sounds are either present, absent, hypoactive, hyperactive for documentation during this exam however, for the outcome it is best when written as follows, "The patient will have active bowel sounds in all four quadrants during the pcs."

✗ **Saying "patient will demonstrate increased tolerance" for an Activity intolerance outcome.** For Activity intolerance, you need to focus on the activity and the intolerance in the outcome so how will they demonstrate an increased tolerance? We usually focus on shortness of breath on exertion or weakness. What do you expect to see?

Be specific. An example would be, "The patient will ambulate with no shortness of breath during the pcs." Ambulation is the activity and shortness of breath is the intolerance that you don't want to see.

✗ Encouraging fluids for Impaired gas exchange or for Ineffective breathing pattern. Interventions should be what you are assigned and it is also wise if you find them in the intervention section of your care plan book. If the interventions are not in your care plan book, you must be prepared to explain how that intervention moves the patient toward the outcome. Encouraging fluids helps loosen secretions so that they can be expelled which is a better intervention for Ineffective airway clearance.

✗ Focusing on lung sounds as an outcome for Ineffective breathing pattern. The outcome idea should also come from your Mosby's or care plan book. If the examiner says 'show me where you got this outcome' and you cannot, it is their discretion to pass or fail you on the decision you made to use that outcome. Having clear lung sounds is not an outcome option in Mosby's for Ineffective breathing pattern.

✗ Saying lung sounds will be "clearer" during pcs. The outcome has to be clear and measurable. How do you measure "clearer?" The lung sounds are either clear or abnormal. The outcome would be, "The patient will have clear lung sounds in upper and lower lobes bilaterally during the pcs."

✗ Using a gait belt as an intervention for mobility. When mobility is assigned on your pcs assignment, it will be specified to what assistive devices you are to use so if a gait belt is not on your pcs assignment, you do not use that as an intervention. Follow the instructions and do only what you are told to do.

✗ **Using "incentive spirometry" as an intervention for Ineffective breathing pattern.** Incentive spirometry is not a listed intervention in Mosby's for Ineffective breathing pattern. You will have to be able to answer how an incentive spirometer will directly affect the breathing pattern in the box below on your plan of care form.

✗ **Using "incentive spirometry" as an intervention for Ineffective peripheral tissue perfusion.** Incentive spirometry is not listed as an intervention in Mosby's for Ineffective peripheral tissue perfusion. The goal of the I/S is to open the alveoli in order to promote effective gas exchange but when there is a perfusion issue going on, there is no guarantee that any gas exchange will occur in the periphery because of a possible perfusion blockage therefore not making this intervention valid for this Nanda.

✗ **Using sequential compression devices for Impaired gas exchange.** This is very similar to the above common mistake but in reverse. Sequential compression devices are to promote blood flow and prevent blood clotting so that the blood flow will make it back to the heart and lungs to be recirculated and become re-oxygenated. In the periphery, the blood is becoming deoxygenated and not contributing to gas exchange directly. Getting the blood back up to the heart and lungs is very important but is not a direct intervention to help the patient achieve better gas exchange.

Common Care Plans

While there are many Nanda labels to choose from there are about 20 of them that are the most common. I have already given you my top ten choices previously in this study guide but I want to highlight some of the ones that EC students tend to use more than others. Keep in mind that when it comes to Nanda labels it is ok to use the same Nanda over and over on all three of your patients so it's a good idea to be familiar with the most reoccurring ones. Here we will focus on five of the top Nanda labels I strongly encourage you to get more comfortable writing.

Ineffective airway clearance

Remember always to read the definition of the Nanda. Basically this Nanda is used when the patient has some retained secretions and they are unable to clear them. Being unable to clear them could be a positioning issue like having to lay completely flat due to traction or maybe they have a weak cough because they are reluctant due to pain or location of incision or simply their throat is sore from being intubated.

There a multiple reasons you could use this Nanda. The defining characteristics, or the signs and symptoms, you need to read about in the chart or on your patient care assignment to know you are heading in the right direction would be abnormal lung sounds of some kind or weak cough.

It is very important to know if you are assigned interventions that can fix the problem. When you are looking at this problem, the intervention you would want to be assigned would be respiratory management with incentive spirometry or cough and deep breathing exercises because those are designed to clear the airway. I/S and cough and deep breathing exercises are two separate interventions so split them up. When you are only assigned one of those, you will need to come up with another intervention.

Here are some interventions to help the patient have clear lung sounds or have an effective cough:

- I/S
- Cough and deep breathe
- Position upright
- Encourage fluids
- Inhaler (if assigned)
- Expectorant (if assigned)

This is how your care plan could look:

---

1. Rhonchi in bases

2. Shortness of breath

Ineffective airway clearance

Rationale: A clear airway is essential for proper oxygenation. If Mr. _____ continues to have retained secretions, it places him at risk for pneumonia and atelectasis.

Related factor: Retained secretions

Outcome: The patient will have clear lung sounds in upper and lower lobes bilaterally after interventions x 1 during pcs

Intervention #1: Encourage patient to perform I/S x 5

[promotes movement of secretions, opens the alveoli, promoting gas exchange]

Intervention #2: Encourage patient to cough and deep breathe

[enhances removal of secretions]

The outcome is very specific. The outcome is patient centered so it always begins with "the patient will" then it tells what you want them to do which is have clear breath sounds and where you want them. I preferably want no abnormal breath sounds anywhere at any time but especially don't want them after I perform the interventions that are supposed to fix the problem.

One of the most common mistakes I see with this care plan is for an intervention students will put "administer oxygen." Although oxygen is great for improving gas exchange, if there is a restricted airway then oxygen is not going to help and oxygen definitely does not clear the breath sounds so it is not an appropriate intervention for this Nanda.

For an outcome, do not say the patient will "maintain" a patent airway or will "maintain" clear lung sounds because maintain means you are already doing it and you only have a risk for care plan. You can use maintain as an intervention to continue treatment of something like IV fluids or oxygen. Interventions cannot be collaborative. This means using other ancillary departments to perform the interventions in not acceptable. For example, you would not write an intervention to have respiratory therapy to administer a nebulizer treatment or you would not write an intervention for any referrals to an outside community resource.. This is where care plan rules vary from school to school or facilities.

Impaired Gas Exchange

When you see this Nanda, I want you to think about oxygen being a "gas" and if you are assigned oxygen management then that is a pretty good indicator that this would be a good Nanda to use. Most of the time the cause of the Impaired gas exchange is usually ventilation perfusion imbalance or alveolar capillary membrane changes. It could be a medical diagnosis of asthma,

COPD, pneumonia, bronchitis, etc, but all of those diagnoses refer back to ventilation perfusion imbalance. The aeb or signs and symptoms would be fluctuations in oxygen saturations, abnormal breathing, confusion, nasal flaring.

What you will want to assess will depend on your outcome. A common outcome is that the patient will have O2 sats of 95% or greater while on 2lpm NC. Always put whether they are on room air or O2 and be specific how much. If that is your outcome then your assessment will be to monitor O2 saturations via pulse oximetry, though you must be assigned to do this.

Possible interventions for this Nanda that will help to get those O2 sats up:

- Position upright
- Maintain O2 at _____lpm via _____(route)
- Encourage slow deep breaths
- Deep breathing and coughing (if assigned resp. mgmt.)
- I/S times however many repetitions you are assigned (is often not an intervention in your Mosby's book for this Nanda so be careful and be able to explain it)

A common mistake made by students is using an outcome or assessment that focuses on arterial blood gases. Blood gases are not the same as oxygen saturations. I know you might laugh at this thinking that someone should know the difference but there are students who do not know the difference. You will not be interpreting blood gases nor will you be using them in your outcome statement or validation assessment.

Assessments:

1. O2 sats 92%

2. Short of breath

Impaired gas exchange

Rationale: Gas exchange is essential to provide oxygen to all of the tissues of the body and if Mr. _____ does not have proper gas exchange, it can lead to hypoxia, confusion, and ischemia.

Related factor: Ventilation perfusion imbalance

Outcome: The patient will demonstrate adequate oxygenation by having O2 saturations of 95% or greater while on _____ (room air? Or ___lpm O2) during the pcs

Intervention #1: position upright

[facilitates better lung expansion promoting better gas exchange]

Intervention #2: administer O2 via 2lpm NC

[provides supplemental oxygen in aide in increased oxygenation]

Impaired Comfort

When a patient is uncomfortable, it can be for various reasons. This Nanda is used when you think that something could be causing the patient discomfort. It could be itching, nausea, unfamiliar environment, too cold, too hot, etc.

You choose this Nanda when you are specifically assigned comfort management because you already know that critical elements for that assignment requires you to perform at least two comfort measures. Those comfort measures should be your interventions that you are already going to do. You would not use pain relief measures for interventions so it is up to you to know the difference between the them.

There is no related factor section for this Nanda because the related factors are too numerous to list. It would have to be specific to your patient on what is causing the discomfort.

This is how your care plan could look:

Assessments:

1. Verbalizes 'can't get comfortable in bed'

2. Restless

Impaired comfort

Rationale: Being comfortable promotes compliance with care as well as healing. If Mr. Smith is not comfortable, he might not be willing to participate in his care placing him at risk for immobility, delayed wound healing, and increases his risk for DVTs and pneumonia.

Related factor: prolonged bedrest/can't reposition self/ unfamiliar environment

Outcome: The patient will verbalize being more comfortable after interventions during pcs (is always better if you know a specific thing that is making them uncomfortable like itching... then you would say the patient will verbalize that itching has improved....the more specific the better)

Intervention #1: reposition patient x1

[relieves pressure off specific areas promoting comfort]

Intervention #2: straighten linens

[removing wrinkles in linens can make the patient more comfortable as well as prevent additional skin breakdown]

Ineffective Peripheral Tissue Perfusion

This Nanda is used when you are assigned a peripheral neurovascular management and when the patient has a decrease in blood circulation. Often the cause is diabetes, smoking, hypertension, tissue trauma, and immobility but not limited to just these. The signs and symptoms you would expect to see in the chart or hear from the nurse prior to seeing the patient would be weak pulses, cool extremities, capillary refill greater than three seconds, altered sensation, discoloration, or delayed peripheral wound healing.

One of the common problems I see when grading this type of care plan is that the student leaves off the word peripheral when writing the Nanda label or they are not specific enough on their assessment and outcomes.

This is how your care plan could look:

Assessments:

1. Weak bilateral lower extremity pulses

2. Cool lower extremities

Ineffective peripheral tissue perfusion

Rationale: Tissue perfusion is essential to provide blood flow, nutrients, and oxygen to the tissues of the body. When perfusion is impaired it places Mr. Smith at risk for DVTs, delayed wound healing, possible necrosis and infection or amputation of the limbs

Related factor: Diabetes

Outcome: The patient will have palpable strong and equal bilateral pedal pulses during pcs

Intervention #1: Provide sequential compression devices while in bed

[sequential compression devices provide a regulation of blood flow to the extremities]

Intervention #2: Ambulate in room x 1

[Ambulation aids in promoting circulation throughout the body]

Other possible interventions could be

- Blanket for warmth
- Elevation of an edematous extremity (when venous)
- Apply compression stockings
- Administer Heparin, Coumadin, lovenox

Ineffective Breathing Pattern

This Nanda is about the patient not breathing normally. They are either breathing too slow, too fast, working to breathe, breathing shallow, or anything abnormal with inspiration or expiration.

Other interventions could be:

- Encourage pursed lip breathing
- Encourage patient to sit up right or lean over a table
- Provide a fan
- Schedule rest periods
- Provide small frequent meals

Assessments:

1. Nasal flaring

2. Tachypnea

Ineffective Breathing Pattern

Rationale: Being able to breathe comfortably promotes ability to participate in care. If Mr. Smith cannot participate in care, it can lead to immobility which increase the risk for pneumonia, atelectasis, and DVTs.

Related factor: musculoskeletal impairment, neurological impairment, neuromuscular impairment

Outcome: The patient will have even and unlabored respirations during pcs or after interventions (or the patient will report ability to breathe comfortably)

Intervention #1: Administer O2 (as ordered...be specific)

[supplemental O2 can lessen the body's increased workload required to maintain oxygen saturation levels]

Intervention #2: Encourage deep breaths at intervals

[Encouraging deep breaths at intervals can help slow down the respirations to prevent dizziness and hyperventilation]

Activity Intolerance

As the words imply, the patient becomes extremely short of breath or fatigued during normal activity. The level of shortness of breath or fatigue seems disproportionate to the activity level.

Common causes:

- Heart failure
- Myocardial infarction
- Prolonged bedrest
- General deconditioning

Assessments:

1. shortness of breath with ambulation

2. complains of weakness

Activity Intolerance

Rationale: Being able to participate in activity enhances blood flow, encourages patient to participate in care and prevents deconditioning, pneumonia, atelectasis, DVTs....

Related factor: bedrest, generalized weakness, imbalance between oxygen supply and demand (pick one)

Outcome: Patient will ambulate with no shortness of breath after interventions

Intervention #1: Assist with ambulation

[Assisting will help the patient pace themselves reducing exertion and shortness of breath]

Intervention #2: Provide rest periods

[This will allow for prevention of air hunger, to help with exertion]

Hint: The nursing student may see an order on the assignment to ambulate with assistance – but it is not due to a true "mobility" problem. It is related to the patient's inability to tolerate activity.

Other possible interventions:

- Range of motion exercises
- Emotional support
- Conscious controlled breathing
- Slow the pace of care
- Assistive devices
- Administer oxygen

Impaired Physical Mobility

As the words imply, this diagnosis is most appropriate for a patient who is primarily on bedrest, not yet ambulatory, and may not even be able to sit up in a chair. The patient clearly has difficulty repositioning self in the bed.

Common causes:

- Spine or hip surgery or other orthopedic surgeries
- Stroke
- Paraplegia
- Dementia or other neurological disorders (MS, ALS, etc.)
- Cast on limb
- Needs crutches, walker, wheelchair
- Amputation/missing limbs
- Arthritis

Assessments:

1. Unsteady gait

2. Walks stooped over

Impaired Physical Mobility

Rationale: Mr. Smith needs to be mobile to prevent deconditioning which can lead to further complications such as contractures, DVTs, and pneumonia

Related factor: decreased muscle strength, musculoskeletal impairment, reconditioning, tissue trauma, reluctance to initiate movement (pick one)

Outcome: The patient will ambulate with a steady gait after interventions during the pcs

Intervention #1: Provide walker, crutches, cane (when prescribed)

[These items allow for stabilization when ambulating]

Intervention #2: Treat pain before ambulating (when ordered)

[Treating pain will allow the patient to ambulate with more comfort and therefore more willing to ambulate and prevent deconditioning]

Example for "Impaired physical mobility."

- AEB: "Patient has an unsteady gait while ambulating to bathroom."
- Assessment: "Assess patient's gait while ambulating to bathroom"

Sample outcome:

- "Patient will have a steady gait while ambulating to bathroom."

Impaired Physical Mobility vs Activity Intolerance

These two diagnoses are often confused.

Look at the patient's signs and symptoms, as well as the medical history, to determine which one is most appropriate.

- Does the patient have some kind of difficulty moving the extremities? Then you are looking at "Impaired physical mobility." (It's all about the "mobility.")
- Does the patient become extremely short of breath during mild activity, such as showering, dressing, or short walks? Then you are looking at "Activity intolerance." (It's all about the "activity.")

Dysfunctional Gastrointestinal Motility

The focus on this Nanda is all about the gut and motility. Whenever there is a problem with the movement of the bowels whether increased, decreases or lack of peristalsis.

Other interventions:

Assessments:

1. abdominal distention

2. hypoactive bowel sounds

Dysfunctional Gastrointestinal Motility

Rationale: It is important for proper gastric motility to allow for proper digestion of nutrients and promoting healing. If this does not occur, Mr. Smith is at risk for ileus, impaction, rupture/perforation, and sepsis (peritonitis)

Related factor: Immobility, malnutrition, tissue trauma, treatment regimen (like narcotics) *pick only one

Outcome: The patient will have active bowel sounds in all four quadrants during the pcs

Intervention #1: Administer colace, protonix, etc...(but only one)

[providing medications will encourage proper digestion of nutrients as well as stimulation of gastric secretions promoting peristalsis]

Intervention #2: Ambulate in room x 1

[Ambulation aids in promoting circulation throughout the body and enhancing peristalsis]

This particular Nanda has very few interventions. Medications and Ambulation along with diet/nutrition are the 3 main interventions.

Care Plan Practice

Male with adenocarcinoma, Left chest portacath,

Safety: Side rails up x 2; allergic to iodine and quinine

Musculoskeletal Management: Bedrest with bathroom privileges (assist with 1 or 2 persons) and reposition x 1

Vital Signs: Tympanic temp, apical HR, RR, manual BP, 0-10 pain scale

Fluid management: 900 ml fluid restriction, low sodium diet, lean meat, boost with meals

Respiratory Management with O2 sats and notify if sats are <92, I/S x5, Deep breathe and cough

O2 Management and patient is on 2.5 liters via NC

0900 Meds: Protonix, metoprolol, ASA, Vit B, Vit C, Vit E, zinc, MVI, spironolactone

From the chart:

Hx of CHF, pleural effusion, pericardial effusion

shortness of breath on exertion

Rhonchi in the bases

From the primary nurse:

Fall risk

Complains of weakness

O2 sats are 93%

Edema to the lower extremities

Practice Assignment 1

Follow the mnemonic MAMM. Following MAMM is to help you brainstorm all possible Nanda labels. Once we come up with a list of Nanda labels, we will prioritize according to Maslow to see which one is the top pick. If you are writing a GRID it is best you go ahead and write your GRID out prior to beginning to write the care plans. Look at your managements first.

You have oxygen management, ask yourself, does this patient have an actual problem? If no, move to your next assignment. If yes, now we find a Nanda label. In this situation, yes they do have a problem. They are on oxygen and have CHF, pleural effusion and shortness of breath.

What possible Nanda labels go with oxygen management?

- Impaired gas exchange
- Ineffective breathing pattern
- Activity intolerance

Out of your options of Nanda labels, until you know for sure where you would like to go, look up each and every one of them and read the definition to determine which care plan you would like to write. I have chosen Impaired gas exchange because first thing I think of is that oxygen is a "gas" and the Nanda Impaired Gas Exchange matches up. But I am not sure that this will be my main focus so lets keep brainstorming all possible Nanda labels.

Next I look at respiratory management. I ask myself if they have a problem and according to the chart, there is rhonchi in the bases so yes they have a problem. Now I have to find out what Nanda labels will go with respiratory management.

The possible Nanda labels are:

- Impaired Gas Exchange
- Ineffective Breathing Pattern
- Ineffective Airway Clearance
- Activity Intolerance

Based on the definitions of each Nanda, I have chosen Ineffective Airway Clearance.

Keep on looking at all of your managements. I am going to look at musculoskeletal management and when I ask if there is a problem, yes. They are weak and a fall risk. So the possible Nandas that go with these problems are:

- Impaired Physical Mobility
- Activity Intolerance

Last but not least, there is fluid management. Ask yourself, do they have a problem? They are on fluid restriction and they need a nutritional supplement so I would say yes.

Possible Nandas for these problems would be:

- Excess fluid volume
- Imbalanced nutriton

Since I am using a GRID, I would list all possible Nandas in one of my blank boxes (usually box 9). So, all possible Nandas for this patient would be:

Impaired Gas Exchange
Ineffective Breathing Pattern
Ineffective Airway Clearance
Activity Intolerance
Impaired Physical Mobility
Excess Fluid Volume
Imbalanced Nutrition

Out of your options of Nanda labels, until you know for sure where you would like to go, look up each and every one of them and read the definition to determine which care plan you would like to write. Now, prioritize according to Maslows to see which would be highest priority.

In the beginning I would suggest working all of the possible Nanda labels/care plans just to get the experience then reason through your priority choice. So here are some examples:

Example care plan 1

Assessments:

1. Shortness of breath on exertion

2. Rhonchi in the bases

Impaired gas exchange

Rationale: Proper gas exchange is necessary to provide oxygen and nutrients to all of the organs in the body. If Mr. Smith does not have proper gas exchange, it places him at risk for hypoxia and confusion and cellular death.

Related factor: alveolar capillary membrane changes

Outcome: The patient will demonstrate adequate oxygenation as evidenced by having O2 sats of 95% or greater while on 2.5 lpm NC during pcs (I got the idea out of Mosby's and matched it to my patient since we are not told to interpret arterial blood gases and you have to say whether the O2 sats are on O2 and how much or on room air)

Intervention #1: Position upright

Rationale: facilitates better lung expansion

Intervention #2: Maintain oxygen via 2lpm NC

Rationale: provides oxygen supplementation to promote better gas exchange

---

Example care plan 2

Assessments:

1. Shortness of breath

2. O2 sats 93%

Ineffective breathing pattern

Rationale: Being able to breathe comfortably promotes ability to participate in care. If Mr. Smith cannot participate in care, it can lead to immobility which increase the risk for pneumonia, atelectasis, and DVTs.

Related factor: chest wall deformity or musculoskeletal impairment or respiratory muscle fatigue

Outcome: Patient will demonstrate even and unlabored respirations during pcs or Patient will have no shortness of breath during pcs or Patient will report the ability to breathe comfortably during the pcs. (so you have a couple of options to choose from but when using no shortness of breath, you cannot say "less" shortness of breath)

Intervention #1: Position upright

[positioning upright allows for better chest wall expansion]

Intervention #2: Encourage slow deep breaths

[Encouraging deep breaths at intervals can help slow down the respirations to prevent dizziness and hyperventilation]

Example care plan 3

Assessments:

1. Rhonchi in bases

2. O2 sats 93%

Ineffective airway clearance

Rationale: A clear airway is necessary for proper gas exchange. If Mr. Smith does not have a clear airway, it places him at risk for pneumonia and atelectasis

Related factor: retained secretions or respiratory muscle fatigue

Outcome: Patient will demonstrate even and unlabored respirations during pcs or Patient will have no shortness of breath during pcs or Patient will report the ability to breathe comfortably during the pcs. (so you have a couple of options to choose from but when using no shortness of breath, you cannot say "less" shortness of breath)

Intervention #1: I/S x 5

[promotes movement of secretions, opens the alveoli, promoting gas exchange]

Intervention #2: Deep breathing and coughing exercises

[enhances the removal of secretions]

All 3 of these Nanda labels would be correct if the outcome and interventions are written correctly. There are multiple options for your interventions but you keep asking yourself: If I do this intervention, will it move the patient toward the outcome? The answer has to be yes.

For this situation Impaired gas exchange focuses on the O2 sats and Ineffective breathing pattern focuses on the shortness of breath and airway clearance focuses on the lung sounds so those are my pics. The way I look at it is, if I clear the airway first, that will slow down the respirations as well as enhance the gas exchange so my first pick would be Ineffective airway clearance. It does not mean the other two are wrong! This is where your personal experience and knowledge comes into play. Also, don't get discouraged if you don't come up with multiple labels or if you come up with too many labels. It might take you a lot longer to write these at first but you are essentially writing multiple care plans and that is some good practice until you get used to what each Nanda is about.

Practice Assignment 2

Follow MAMM.

Pat (Grady 6/15) 8 yo male with sickle cell in a vaso-occlusive crisis
Safety: side rails up x 2
Musculoskeletal management: OOB x1 with assistance
Fluid Management: Encourage fluids, soft bland diet, IV of D5NS@69 ml/hr on ICD
Peripheral neurovascular management to upper
0845 Meds: Folic acid and Zantac orally
Comfort management: with comfort measures using a 0-10 verbal comfort scale.
From the chart:
Pain is in the back and left hand and patient is rating an 8 at all times
On PCA of morphine
From the nurse:
Upper extremities are cool on the left, pulses are present but weaker in the left
Has decreased strength in left arm
Not talking much
Grimacing

Comfort management, does the patient have a problem? Yes and the label that goes with comfort management is Impaired comfort.

Next management is peripheral neurovascular management. Does the patient have a problem? Yes. Temperature, pulses and strength are a problem. So what Nanda goes with this? Ineffective peripheral tissue perfusion.

Next management is musculoskeletal management. Do they have a problem? They need assistance getting out of bed. So I would say yes but I need more questions answered so this might not be a top pick for me unless I get answers. The Nanda that goes with this would be Impaired physical mobility.

Last management is fluid management. Do they have a problem? We are to encourage fluids and maintain the IV. Could there be a problem? Yes there could be. This might require more thinking critically but with sickle cell crises, they usually are dehydrated or have an infection that led to the crisis. So I would say yes they have Deficient fluid volume. However, I would want to know what their mucous membranes and turgor is doing in order for me to lean more toward this Nanda.

Okay, now I have the following Nandas that I would write in box 9 on my GRID:

- Impaired comfort
- Ineffective peripheral tissue perfusion
- Impaired physical mobility
- Deficient fluid volume

Remember, in the beginning you should really work all the Nandas to familiarize yourself with the specific care plans for them.

Example care plan 1

Assessments:

1. Grimacing

2. Not talking much

Impaired comfort

Rationale: If the patient is comfortable, they are more willing to participate in their care which will enhance healing by promotion of nutrition and circulation. Preventing a prolonged hospital stay and risk for pneumonia.

Related factor: sickle cell crisis

Outcome: The patient will have a comfort rating of 6 or greater on a 0-10 verbal comfort scale after interventions

Intervention #1: Reposition patient

[repositioning provides comfort by getting the patient off of the pressure points]

Intervention #2: Provide TV for distraction

[the ability to focus on something else will take the mind off the current uncomfortable situation]

Example care plan 2

Assessments:

1. Cool left upper extremity

2. Weak left upper extremity

Ineffective peripheral tissue perfusion

Rationale: Tissue perfusion is essential to provide blood and oxygen necessary for the organs to function and to prevent death to the tissues, necrosis, amputation, increased pain, infection.

Related factor: sickle cell crisis

Outcome: The patient will have warm bilateral upper extremities during the pcs

Intervention #1: Assist patient OOB x 1

[movement enhances blood flow throughout the body and prevents deconditioning]

Intervention #2: Provide blanket to upper extremities

[this will provide warmth enhancing blood flow to the affected limbs]

Impaired physical mobility and Deficient fluid volume are not to be ruled out but are not as strong as Impaired comfort and Ineffective peripheral tissue perfusion. Both are good strong care plans. In my mind, if they are not comfortable, they will not get out of bed for you and might refuse other interventions therefore, I would want to focus on the comfort first. You may want to focus on perfusion and that is fine too.

Stephan male with laparoscopic appendectomy yesterday

Safety: side rails up x 2; NKA

Mobility: ambulate from bed to chair

Fluid Management: IV of LR @ 150 ml/hr ICD, clear liquid diet; encourage fluids voids in urinal

Vital Signs: axillary temp, apical HR, RR, manual BP

Comfort management: with comfort measures using a 0-10 verbal comfort scale

Abdominal Assessment

Peripheral Neurovascular Management of the lower

From the chart:

Received dilaudid at 0730

Complaining of nausea and zofran ordered

No gas and no stool

Bowel sounds are hypoactive

From primary nurse

Lower extremities are WNL

guards abdomen

grimaces

Bulky dressing to abdomen

Practice Assignment 3

Follow your MAMM. Comfort management. Does the patient have a problem? Yes they do. The Nanda is Impaired comfort.

Next management is peripheral neurovascular management. Do they have a problem? No. Everything is within normal limits according to the primary nurse so don't dwell on it, answer no and keep moving.

Next management is fluid management. Do they have a problem? Well, we can assume they lost fluids during surgery. We are to encourage fluids and provide IV fluids but I would like to know for sure what the mucous membranes are doing as well as turgor so I might just hold onto this as an option but not be my main focus.

Now we move to assessments and we have abdominal. Do they have a problem? Yes they do and it is more than one problem. The Nanda is Dysfunctional gastrointestinal motility.

Assessments:

1. grimacing

2. guarding abdomen

Impaired comfort

Rationale: If the patient is comfortable, they are more willing to participate in their care which will enhance healing by promotion of nutrition and circulation. Preventing a prolonged hospital stay and risk for pneumonia.

Related factor: tissue trauma

Outcome: The patient will rate comfort a 6 or greater on a 0-10 verbal comfort scale during pcs

Intervention #1: Reposition x 1

[repositioning provides comfort by getting the patient off of the pressure points]

Intervention #2: TV for distraction, conversation, guided imagery, etc.

[the ability to focus on something else will take the mind off the current uncomfortable situation]

Example care plan 1

With no gas, no stool, complains of nausea, here are a couple of Nanda choices dealing with abdominal assessment:

- Dysfunctional gastrointestinal motility
- Nausea
- Deficient fluid volume

Example care plan 2

Assessments:

1. not passing gas

2. nausea

(could also be no stool or hypoactive bowel sounds)

Dysfunctional gastrointestinal motility

Related factor: tissue trauma

Outcome: Patient will pass gas x 1 during pcs OR patient will have soft formed stool x 1 during pcs OR patient will consume clear liquid diet with no complaints of nausea during pcs

Intervention #1: Assist with ambulation ***Wouldn't necessarily work for nausea***

[ambulation enhances peristalsis]

Intervention #2: Encourage clear liquids

[clear liquids will stimulate gastric secretions and peristalsis]

The funny thing about this Nanda label is that there are very few interventions in your care plan book that are actions. So the three interventions that I found that are actions were some sort of mobility whether reposition or ambulate, oral fluids, and a medication that works on motility like protonix.

Assessments:

1. ?

2. ?

Deficient fluid volume

Rationale: Being well hydrated is essential for all organs to function properly. Mr. Smith lost fluids during surgery and needs to replace them for proper healing to prevent further dehydration, weakness, and organ failure.

Related factor: Active fluid volume loss

Outcome: The patient will have non tenting skin turgor during pcs or the patient will have moist mucus membranes during the pcs

Intervention #1: Administer LR @ 150 ml/hr

[providing intravenous fluids promotes hydration and electrolye balance and promotes healing]

Intervention #2: Encourage clear liquids

[Oral ingestion of fluids promotes hydration]

Example care plan 3

When grading Deficient fluid volume care plans, I see students focusing more on the urine output for the outcome and that is okay however, you are already assigned to check the turgor or mucus membranes and the urine output is if they have anything. The patient may go your entire pcs without voiding and that could cost you a revision. Keep it simple. When your child is dehydrated, how do you know? Sunken eyes, weak, dry mucus membranes. Do you sit there and wonder how many times your child has voided? To me it is not the most obvious observation for deficient fluid volume. Another outcome I see students use is the one about the patient having "normal blood pressure, pulse, and body temperature" but what is normal? You have to be specific.

Finally go to your mobility. Do they have a mobility problem? Maybe, but don't know for sure so a mobility care plan would not be a strong one to use at this point but you do have some other strong ones that would be a priority. And then the last M which is medications, and there are none in this scenario so you leave that alone.

Do you see how I don't have any assessment findings? There was nothing given to me about turgor or mucous membranes. I have a solid care plan if I could just find out that information. So when you are testing, this should trigger your critical thinking skills to find out that information. If you do not find out that information, you cannot write a care plan on what you do not know is an actual problem.

When grading Deficient fluid volume care plans, I see students focusing more on the urine output for the outcome however, you are already assigned to check the turgor or mucus membranes and the urine output is if they have anything. The patient may go your entire pcs without voiding and that could cost you a revision. Keep it simple. When your child is dehydrated, how do you know? Sunken eyes, weak, dry mucus membranes. Do you sit there and wonder how many times your child has voided? Usually not on an hourly basis. To me it is not the most obvious observation for deficient fluid volume. Another outcome I see students use is the one about the patient having "normal blood pressure, pulse, and body temperature" but what is normal? You have to be specific and actually, when are you checking vital signs? Are you going to go back and re-check vital signs at the end of your pcs? Probably not and you can mess yourself up by adding something that you aren't normally doing.

Practice Assignment 4

Amber 78 yo female with history of CVA several years ago, and CHF. Admitted with hyponatremia, lower extremity weakness and SIADH.

Safety: Siderails up x 2, NKA

Vital Signs: HR apical, RR, Oral Temp, manual BP, 0-10 pain scale

Fluid Management: Intake only: fluid restricted to fluids on tray only, regular diet, no IV now (possible order for one tomorrow)

0900 Meds: ASA, Imdur, Protonix, Valsartin

Neurological Assessment

Musculoskeletal Management with AROM to right lower and PROM to left lower reposition x 1

From chart:

Stage II pressure ulcer on buttocks

Weak left side

Lung sounds are clear

Shallow respirations

From nurse:

Occasional confusion to place and time

Wears depends and is incontinent

Rating pain a 2

Here we go. Look at your management first. You have musculoskeletal management. Do they have an issue with movement? They do have lower extremity weakness, yes they do. There are two labels specifically to this. We are going to go ahead and look at mobility at the same time because the labels go with both of these categories. The two specific labels are:

- Impaired bed mobility
- Activity intolerance

Impaired physical mobility would not work here because that label is for when they get out of bed. So when the patient is on bedrest you use Impaired bed mobility

Example care plan 1

Assessments:

1. Weak left side

2. Unable to reposition self

Impaired bed mobility

Rationale: Being mobile is important in circulation and healing. Ms. Smith is compromised due to her CVA, age, incontinence which places her at greater risk of worsening the current skin break down or even more as well as DVTs and pneumonia

Related factor: Insufficient muscle strength, CVA, alteration in cognitive function (pick one)

Outcome: Patient will demonstrate the ability to assist with repositioning by using right side of her body x1 during pcs OR patient will participate with repositioning x 1 during pcs OR patient will demonstrate the ability to direct others on how to do bed positioning (but with the confusion, this one may be harder)

Intervention #1: Assist with repositioning

[this ensures the patient gets moved correctly and provides support until she is strong enough to do it herself]

Intervention #2: AROM to right lower or PROM to left lower

[helps to strengthen the lower extremities so the patient can help to reposition]

Impaired bed mobility is an awkward care plan to write with regards to the outcome but with more practice and understanding of the Nanda, it will feel a little less awkward when writing.

Example care plan 2

Assessments:

1. lower extremity weakness

2. confusion

Activity intolerance

Rationale: Being able to participate with activity allows for better function of all systems. If Ms. Smith is unable to tolerate activity this increases the risk of other complications like DVTs, pneumonia, and deconditioning.

Related factor: generalized weakness, CHF (pick one and you may come up with others)

Outcome: Patient will verbalize increased strength during pcs or patient will participate in repositioning with no complaints of weakness or shortness of breath during pcs (but pick only one)

Intervention #1: Assist with repositioning

[this allows patient to tolerate because they are not having to do it on their own]

Intervention #2: Encourage patient to perform AROM to the lower extremities

could do rest periods, PROM, essentially similar to Impaired bed mobility

[this helps strengthen the patient so that she can tolerate repositioning to prevent complications]

With activity intolerance, students often want to focus on fatigue. If you are being drawn to fatigue, that is an actual Nanda-I label so you may want to look that up and try to work it. Remember to always read the definition prior to formulating your care plan.

Now move onto your assessment. You are assigned neurological assessment. Does your patient have a problem? Yes. They have occasional confusion. The one Nanda that goes with this assessment is acute confusion. And this is really the only one that goes with the neurological assessment. Confusion is either acute or chronic and I am choosing acute because I am assuming it is under 6 months however, when testing, wouldn't that be a great question to ask?

Example care plan 3

Assessments:

1. occasional confusion to place

2. occasional confusion to time

Acute confusion

Rationale: When the patient is confused, they can become anxious and not want to participate in their care. This can prevent complications with not wanting to eat, move, and withdrawal increasing the risk of pneumonia, DVTs, and delayed wound healing

Related factor: age or SIADH or electrolyte imbalance

Outcome: Patient will be oriented to person, place, and time during pcs (pick one)

Intervention #1: Provide reality orientation [this helps re-orient patient]

Intervention #2: Explain routines and procedures in a slow and simple manner [this helps orient and allow patient to process the information to participate]

Other interventions could be use gentle, caring communication or establish a calm environment

Did you notice how the assignment told you the patient was incontinent and had pressure ulcers, also rating pain a 2? Did your mind want to wander there with a skin or tissue integrity problem or pain? You don't want to go there because you were not assigned skin assessment, pain management, or comfort management. Care plans are to be based on your assigned areas of care.

Dani peds substitute 20 yo male with dx of acute pancreatitis, obese/diabetic. Went to ICU 5 days ago and was intubated. Extubated 2 days ago and went to med-surg floor

Fluid Management: Intake only, 2000 cal. ADA diet, fluid ad lib

Respiratory Management DB& Cough and Incentive x 5 repetitions

Abdominal Assessment

Musculoskeletal management: Reposition x1

Meds @ 0900: nexium, lopid, and glucerna shake at 9am

Vital Signs: Apical HR, RR, Ax. Temp, manual BP, pain assessment 0-10 scale and is rating pain a 3

From chart:

Abdomen is distended

Bowel sounds are hypoactive

From nurse:

New onset diabetic

Breath sounds are abnormal (rhonchi)

Getting respiratory treatments and is decreased in the bases

On room air

Practice Assignment 5

Following MAMM, your managements are Respiratory, Musculoskeletal and Fluid. There is really no indicator that there is a Deficient fluid volume issue. There is not indicators that they cannot reposition. What about respiratory? Does the patient have an actual problem? Yes. What Nanda labels go with this management?

- Ineffective airway clearance
- Impaired gas exchange
- Ineffective breathing pattern

Example care plan 1

Assessments:
1. Rhonchi
2. Decreased lung sounds in bases
Ineffective airway clearance Rationale: A clear airway is essential for proper gas exchange. If the airway is not clear, it increases the risk for pneumonia and atelectasis.
Related factor: retained secretions
Outcome: Patient will have clear lung sounds in upper and lower lobes bilaterally after interventions during pcs
Intervention #1: Encourage patient to deep breathe and cough [this aids in the removal of secretions]
Intervention #2: Encourage patient to perform I/S x 5 repetitions
[this also aids in removal of secretions and opening the alveoli for proper gas exchange]

Example care plan 2

Assessments:

1. Rhonchi

2. Decreased lung sounds in bases

Impaired gas exchange

Rationale: A clear airway is essential for proper gas exchange. If the airway is not clear, it increases the risk for pneumonia and atelectasis.

Related factor: alveolar capillary membrane changes

Outcome: Patient will have clear breath sounds in upper and lower lobes bilaterally after interventions during the pcs

Intervention #1: Encourage patient to deep breathe and cough [this aids in the removal of secretions]

Intervention #2: Encourage patient to perform I/S [this also aids in removal of secretions and opening the alveoli for proper gas exchange]

Example care plan 3

Let's take a look at Ineffective breathing pattern.

Assessments:
1. ?
2. ?
Ineffective breathing pattern (r/t respiratory muscle fatigue aeb?)
Rationale:
Related factor: respiratory muscle fatigue
Outcome: Patient will have even and unlabored respirations during pcs or patient will report ability to breath comfortably during pcs
Intervention #1: Encourage patient to deep breathe and cough
Intervention #2: Encourage patient to perform I/S x 5 (but this is not an intervention in my Mosby's book under this Nanda) [this also aids in removal of secretions and opening the alveoli for proper gas exchange]

All three of these care plans have the same interventions. Ineffective airway clearance and Impaired gas exchange have the same outcomes. You could not focus on O2 sats for gas exchange because they said the patient is on room air and they do not give you their O2 sat readings. Now, with the ineffective breathing pattern, there is nothing giving us an indicator that they are having breathing difficulties like tachypnea or dyspnea so until you look into the chart or ask the primary nurse about this, it is not as safe to focus on this label as it would be the other two.

Where do we look next? You guessed it! The assessments and you are assigned abdominal assessment. Does the patient have a problem with this area? Yes. The label that goes with this is Dysfunctional gastrointestinal motility.

Example care plan 4

1. Abdomen distended

2. Hypoactive bowel sounds

Dysfunctional gastrointestinal motility

Rationale: Gastric motility is important to provide nutrients through absorption to all the organs and prevent an ileus, impaction, rupture, and peritonitis.

Related factor: pancreatitis

Outcome: Patient will be free from abdominal distention during pcs or patient will have active bowel sounds in all four quadrants during pcs

Intervention #1 Reposition x 1

[movement of any kind aids in peristaltic activity]

Intervention #2 Administer Nexium

[aids with the gastric acids to stimulate peristalsis]

Other interventions: provide glucerna, offer fluids

After looking at the managements and assessments, you then look at your mobility and medications. In this situation, we have already utilized the Nexium and there are no specific indicators that there is a mobility problem to create a care plan with.

Have you noticed a rhythm or a pattern? These assignments were designed to show you how to think fast and simple with regards to your assignments. I am sure there are other care plan options for these patients, however, if you follow the rules to care planning and keeping it real simple, this will help you be very successful in the planning phase.

Conclusion

Hopefully by now you feel like you have a firm grasp on the concept of writing care plans for your clinical weekend. Keep in mind that these tips and guidelines on writing care plans are specific to Excelsior College's Clinical Performance Nursing Examination. When you work within different healthcare organizations you will need to adjust your care planning to reflect the guidelines that they have set in place. The goal for this book though is to get you through the CPNE®, which if you follow what I have talked about, I'm sure you'll have no problems with.

Instead of just going through the motions and a mental checklist of a care plan though, it will help you to remember *why* you are doing it. Care plans teach nursing students how to think critically and how to care for patients on a more personal level. They help teach how to prioritize care and interventions.

While you might not enjoy writing care plans right now, they are a necessary evil of nursing school. They teach future nurses not just to provide care, but how to provide care that will improve the client's health status. Try not to think of care plans as a menial task that is just required for your test. Instead ask yourself, "what can I do based on what I am assigned to give this patient the best possible care?" If you put the focus on caring for the patient instead of memorizing how to write the formal document, it will help you think logically during your exam which means you'll be writing passing care plans every time.

As you write more care plans your skills for thinking critically and processing information like a professional Registered Nurse will become second nature. You may even come to enjoy writing them, or at least come to appreciate the value of them. Getting comfortable with care planning is just going to take practice though... and a lot of it.

I highly suggest you join a care plan course to perfect your care plan skills from home. Just make sure the course is specific to the CPNE® and reflects all the updates for the current EC Study Guide edition. Finding a care plan course that suits your learning style and having someone critique your assignments will be the most effective way to know what your weaknesses are and how to tighten them up before it comes time for you to test.

I'd like to leave you with these final words.

Never give up.

Cliche, I know, but it's true. We all know this exam is seriously difficult and is a lot of pressure on you. The key is preparation, attitude and diligence. Stay positive and take studying for this exam one bite at a time. Take some time to chew on what you've learned about care plans, practice them, get good at them and *then* bite off your next studying challenge.

If you stand their staring at your 500 page EC study guide thinking, "how the heck am I going to learn *all* this information," or "I'll never be able to memorize *all* this stuff in time," then you're setting yourself up for a lot of undo stress. Start with what you feel your biggest weakness is and work through that before you move on.

I know you can do this. I've helped thousands of students pass the CPNE® and every single one of them was where you are right now. I haven't met a single student that wasn't stressed about this exam so don't beat yourself up for feeling overwhelmed. Just take it one step at a time and soon you'll be able to hold up those CPNE® pass papers.

Good luck on your CPNE®, future RN!

You're closer to passing than you think.

About the Author

Sheri Taylor-Jenkins, RN-C, MSN, has an unparalleled passion for teaching that she has used to help over 4,000 students pass the CPNE® since 2004. Sheri owns and operates ATL Clinical Workshop, the nation's most trusted name in hands-on and online CPNE® preparation.

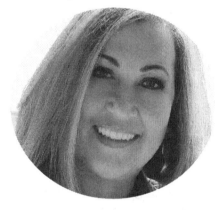

With 27 years as a nurse Sheri's accomplished career boasts such accolades as: Assistant Director, Director, Clinical Coordinator, and Transport Coordinator. For ten years Sheri was also an educator with The American Heart Association in BLS, PALS, NRP, and ACLS as well as a S.T.A.B.L.E. instructor. She has served on multiple committees for JCAHO: policies and procedures, infectious diseases, & quality assurance.

Sheri's first love in nursing is caring for children from birth to 18 years old and she holds national certifications in Neonatal Intensive Care, Low Risk Neonatal, and Maternal Newborn. She enjoys specializing in NICU, PICU, Peds, Peds ER, Peds Psych (particularly autism), and Peds Oncology. She has been lucky enough to work in these specialities at some of the best children's hospitals in the southeast: Children's Healthcare of Atlanta (Scottish Rite, Eggleston, and Hughes Spalding Children's Hospital) and St. Jude's.

Sheri has been nominated as Nurse of the Year by both Southern Regional Medical Center and the Atlanta Journal-Constitution and has authored and co-authored several books and articles, which have appeared in various well respected nursing publications. Sheri holds her Master's Degree in Nursing Education and her Bachelor's in Business Management and now working on her Doctor of Naturopath degree.

Other affiliations include: National Association of Neonatal Nurses Georgia Association of Neonatal Nurses American Nursing Association National Association of Professional Women Association of Perioperative Registered Nurses Cambridge Who's Who Among Professionals National Nurses in Business Association.

Don't Stop Now!

Passing your CPNE® is about to get a whole lot easier!

Want to continue studying for the CPNE® from home? With ATL Clinical's Online CPNE® Workshop you can have instant, unlimited access to over 50 hours of organized video lecture and demonstration proven to double your chances of passing the CPNE®. It's like getting an entire CPNE® workshop from the comfort of your living room!

If you learn better visually and through repetition then our online workshop, *without a doubt*, is the most effective way to study for the CPNE® from home. Accessible 24 hours a day, 7 days a week, you will be able to log into your members area from anywhere you have an internet connection to study videos and demonstrations covering;

- Patient care
- Skills stations
- Careplans
- Medications
- Documentation
- Plus so much more...

Plus, with two care plan homework assignments every week to submit back for grading, you will have the opportunity to have a team of expert CPNE® educators critique your care plans.

There is no way you will go to the CPNE® being anything short of a careplan ninja.

We surveyed over 1,000 previous members (through an *independent*, *unbiased* survey company) and 99.8% say our online CPNE® workshop is a "Must-have to pass the CPNE®!"

Want to join us online?

If you're ready to join the online workshop just go to the website below. We look forward to helping you in the members area!

www.atlclinicalworkshop.com/online-cpne-workshop

Made in the USA
Columbia, SC
08 September 2019